The Parent's Success Guide™ to Organizing

Edited by H. Dismore

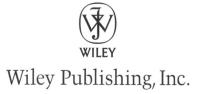

WILEY

Wiley Publishing, Inc.

The Parent's Success Guide™ to Organizing

Published by
Wiley Publishing, Inc.
111 River St.
Hoboken, NJ 07030-5774
www.wiley.com

For general information on our other products and services or to obtain technical support, please contact our Customer Care Department within the U.S. at 800-762-2974, outside the U.S. at 317-572-3993, or fax 317-572-4002.

Wiley also publishes its books in a variety of electronic formats. Some content that appears in print may not be available in electronic books.

Library of Congress Control Number: 2003114884

ISBN: 0-7645-5928-1

Manufactured in the United States of America

10 9 8 7 6 5 4

WILEY

About the Authors

Through her company Everything in Its Place, **Eileen Roth,** co-author of *Organizing For Dummies*, consults with clients including Fortune 500 companies, trade associations, entrepreneurs, and busy individuals and families. Her success shaping up even the organizationally impaired has landed her spots on *Oprah;* the *Today* show with Bryant Gumbel; *Handy Ma'am* with Bev DeJulio; and NBC, ABC, and WGN News. Eileen's organizing fixes have been featured by the *Chicago Tribune* and *Chicago Sun-Times* and on a number of radio stations, and she uses her advanced time-management skills to squeeze in workshops across the country. She recently moved from her hometown of Chicago to Phoenix, Arizona, to be closer to her college-age daughters. She is a member of the National Association of Professional Organizers (NAPO), National Speakers Association (NSA), and American Society for Training and Development (ASTD).

Elizabeth Miles, co-author of *Organizing For Dummies*, is known to her fans for her user-friendly approach to peak performance on many fronts, Elizabeth offers answers that pop off the page and onto your to-do-now list. She's miles of smiles as she tells you how to tune into success, new-millennium style. With a professional career that's run the gamut from banking on Wall Street to booking rock concerts and developing gourmet recipes, Miles relies on a broad range of experience in making the good life easier for busy people. She puts her graduate degree in ethnomusicology to work with her book and CD series *Tune Your Brain: Using Music to Manage Your Mind, Body, and Mood,* which draws upon the latest neurological and medical research about music's effects on the body and mind to create an applied system for listeners. As creator and host of the dialing "Braintuning Break" radio feature, she's taken her advice to the airwaves and earned listener loyalty over three seasons on the California Classical Network. Miles' popular approaches to achieving potential have been extensively covered in national and international media from *Self* to *Success*, PBS to the BBC, while the *Tune Your Brain* CD series has enjoyed long Top Ten runs on Billboard's classical chart. Miles lectures and consults for organizations such as Kaiser Permanente, the Los Angeles Unified School District, the Young Entrepreneurs' Organization, the Wellness Community, and many more concerned with health, education, and performance. As a previously self-professed organizational dummy, she enjoyed applying her trademark knack for making things easy to Eileen's expertise and proven techniques to help bring *Organizing For Dummies* to life. A native of Madison, Wisconsin, Miles holds a master's degree from the University of California, Los Angeles, and a B.A. from Dartmouth College. She lives in Los Angeles.

Heather Heath Dismore began her career as a well-traveled, highly productive restaurant manager. She left the industry to devote time to her family and her love of writing. In a publishing career spanning over a decade, her work has impacted some 400 titles. Her most recent projects include *Indian Cooking For Dummies*, part of the compilation *Cooking Around the World All-in-One For Dummies*. She holds a B.A. from DePauw University. Dismore resides in Springfield, Missouri, with her husband, who is a professional chef, and their two daughters.

Publisher's Acknowledgments

Some of the people who helped bring this book to market include the following:

Editor: Elizabeth Kuball

Acquisitions Editors: Holly Gastineau-Grimes and Joyce Pepple

Technical Editor: Dorothy Breininger

Cover Photo: © EasyClosets.Com, 2003

Interior Design: Kathie S. Schnorr

Table of Contents

☺ ☻ ☹ ☺ ☻ ☹ ☺ ☻ ☹ ☺ ☻ ☹ ☺ ☻ ☹ ☺ ☻ ☹ ☺

Table of Contents

☺ ☻ ☹ ☺ ☻ ☹ ☺ ☻ ☹ ☺ ☻ ☹ ☺ ☻ ☹ ☺ ☺ ☻ ☹ ☺

Table of Contents

Part 1
Getting Started

Getting organized can seem like an overwhelming task — especially when you're a busy parent, trying to keep your kids, your spouse, your house, and all the other projects in your life organized as well. You are the original multitasker and project manager, whether you know it or not. In this part, you'll discover a few basic systems and tools to organize whatever you need to in your own life.

Chapter 1 outlines the process and introduces the basics of organizing, such as understanding the cost of clutter, dealing with clutter immediately (before it multiplies), and getting your mind in the mode to organize. Chapter 2 gives you the nuts and bolts. It introduces easy systems for classifying the stuff in your life, getting rid of what you really don't need, and putting everything in its P-L-A-C-E.

Chapter 1

The Basics of Organizing

Y ou probably think clutter-busting is going to hurt. For many people, getting organized sounds less appealing — and more complicated — than a trip to the dentist. You may have put off cleaning up your life by figuring that if you're not organized yet, you must have the wrong personality type. Getting organized may seem to go against the grain and only cause pain.

In This Chapter

☺ Calculating the cost of disorganization in dollars and cents

☺ How organizing increases time, productivity, and good health

☺ Stopping clutter-causers in their tracks

Then there are the more specific anti-organization arguments. "I don't have time," say many, mixing up the excuse with the exact reason to do it. Others worry that organization will limit their creativity or rob them of their spark. Some people steer clear because they fear that organizing systems may turn them into uptight rule makers or rigid control freaks.

The techniques in this book provide simple and proven ways to organize your life the way *you* like to live it. Get organized to achieve peak potential and enjoy lifelong peace.

First Things First: Using This Book

This book is part of a series called *The Parent's Success Guide.* Its main purpose is to help you, a busy, multitasking mom (or dad!), make some positive changes in your life as a parent — in a minimum amount of time.

Brought to you by the makers of the world-famous *For Dummies* series, this book provides straightforward advice, hands-on information, and helpful, practical tips — all of it on, about, and for being a smart parent. And this book does so with warmth, encouragement, and gentleness — as a trusted friend would do.

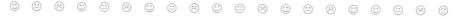

This book isn't meant to be read from front to back, so you don't have to read the entire book to understand what's going on. Just go to the chapter or section that interests you. Keep an eye out for text in *italics*, which indicates a new term and a nearby definition — no need to spend time hunting through a glossary.

While reading this book, you'll see these icons sprinkled here and there:

 This icon points out advice that saves time, requires less effort, achieves a quick result, or helps make a task easier.

 This icon signifies information that's important to keep in mind.

 This icon alerts you to areas of caution or danger — negative information you need to be aware of.

If you'd like more comprehensive information about a particular subject covered in this book, you may want to pick up a copy of the classic *For Dummies* book covering the same topic. This book consists primarily of text compiled from *Organizing For Dummies*.

Living in an Overstuffed World

Imagine that a tornado hit your house and whisked it away. What would you really need to start over again? What would you truly miss? Many people have to think in these dramatic terms in order to sort out the productive elements from the clutter in their lives.

Why? Because the world is overstuffed. Houses and offices are filled to the brim, and yet advertisers still beg consumers to buy more. Sandwiches get bigger all the time, and people do, too. Cities are bursting at the seams; schools are overcrowded. Society has adopted an overstuffed mentality, and then you wonder why you can't think clearly or feel peaceful and calm.

Getting organized is about *unstuffing* your life, clearing out the deadweight in places from your closet to your calendar to your computer, and then installing systems that keep the good stuff in its place. Organizing is a liberating and enlightening experience that can enhance your effectiveness and lessen your stress every day, and it's all yours simply for saying "No" to clutter.

Clutter happens when you don't put things in place, whether on your desktop, inside the filing cabinet, in your calendar, or atop the kitchen counter. Bringing things into a room and not putting them back where they belong creates clutter. Leaving toys in the hallway, newspapers in the living room, or e-mail in your incoming queue clutters up your space. Unimportant obligations are clutter in the day. Jamming too many things in your home, office, or schedule — filling every space, littering your life — doesn't give you more power or pleasure. Random articles and activities give you clutter. By getting organized with the techniques in this book, you can leave space free to work, play, and be.

Piled-up clutter

Then there's that special form of clutter you may recognize with a guilty smile: the pile. Although making a pile could seem like putting things away, nothing could be farther from the truth. Think about what happens when you make a pile: Now you have to dig through everything on top to find what you need, instead of simply going to the file or drawer or shelf where the item should be. Whether it's papers, toys, clothes, or computer disks, making piles makes work and wastes time.

Mental clutter

The most disorienting form of clutter is mental. Mixing up your mind with commitments you can't keep track of, things you can't find or don't know how to do, or chaotic surroundings can cause stress and block basic cognitive processes. If you have trouble making decisions; if you frequently have to go back to the office, the store, or home to pick up something you left behind; if you're worried that you can't accomplish what's expected or needed, from cooking dinner to finalizing a deal, then you're probably suffering from the confusion caused by mental clutter. When you get organized, you'll gain planning, time-management, and placement techniques to clear your mind and de-stress your life.

The Cost of Clutter

The reason for reading and using this book to organize your life is simple: Clutter of all kinds costs you dearly. The costs of clutter range from hard cash to time, space, health, and your relationships with people. You may be unaware of the price you pay for overstuffing your life, but when you analyze the cost of clutter, the rewards of getting organized become clear.

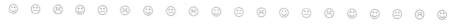

Time

What's the one commodity you can never replace in this life? Time. When it's gone, it's gone. You can't retrieve, relive, or replay a moment of it. Time is the most precious gift, yet people casually throw it away every day. Did you spend time looking for something this morning? Miss an appointment, train, or plane? Drag your way through a report after wasting your peak work time on opening the mail? Maybe you waited in rush-hour traffic because you left too late. Perhaps you lost an hour of relaxation time because getting dinner on and off the table takes too long, your laundry room is set up wrong, or you went to the grocery or office-supply store without a list.

 Every second counts. Getting organized helps you get things done fast so you can spend the extra time enjoying life.

Money

The wallet is often where people feel things first, and disorganization could be draining yours. Consider your own situation, and take a minute to calculate the dollar cost of the clutter in your life based on the following:

* **Rent or mortgage:** All the square feet filled with junk in your home, office, or storage locker

* **Wage or salary:** The time you waste doing things inefficiently, twice, or without a plan, *plus* the raises you haven't received because you're not working at peak potential

* **Overpaid for purchases:** Excess costs from buying at the last minute, from the wrong source, or in the wrong quantity

* **Duplicate purchases:** Cost of things you've bought duplicates of because you couldn't find yours, forgot you had one, or lost the instruction book or warranty to use it or get it fixed

* **Penalties:** Fees, interest, and penalties for late payments and bounced checks

* **Depreciation:** Loss of resale value of cars and other equipment you're not maintaining properly

* **Medical bills:** From doctor's visits to aspirin and stomach medications, all the money you spend because stress is sabotaging your health

Now imagine: What can you do with all that money when you get it back by getting organized?

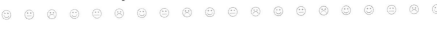

Health

Getting things done when you're disorganized is hard enough, but how about when you're sick, too? Over time, disorganization can actually contribute to disease. Stress can cause disorders from headache and fatigue to ulcers, high blood pressure, even heart disease. Missing checkups or neglecting treatments can allow conditions to get worse. Simply can't make the time to exercise? You could be shaving years off your life.

Space

People today are so accustomed to being crowded that forgetting the value of physical space and letting yours get overstuffed with things you don't want or need is easy to do. Yet space creates appreciation for everything it contains. As they tell you in music class, without the rests, the notes lose all their interest. When you get organized, you can find out how to stop filling up space and let it stay empty, so you have room to breathe, dance, and dream.

Reputation and relationships

Missing birthdays. Blowing deadlines. Greeting guests with a harried face and house. Letting clients, colleagues, and your boss see you surrounded by piles of papers and supplies. What do you think clutter does to your reputation and relationships?

A cluttered home puts your family on edge and discourages guests from having fun or even coming by. High-stress holidays and parties, late or poorly chosen gifts, leaving the kids waiting at soccer practice, forgetting to follow up on a sick relative or pick up your partner's dry cleaning when you promised — all these situations can lessen the love and laughter in your life. Is that a price you're willing to pay?

Getting organized can enhance all your interpersonal relationships by letting your talents shine. Order and clear expectations create a comfortable environment, freeing people up to enjoy and express themselves. Organization can boost self-esteem and the regard in which others hold you. This confidence will reflect in everything you do.

The Causes of Clutter

Clutter is costly but not inevitable — clutter is caused by patterns and practices that you can change. If you have clutter-causing habits, you are not alone. The age of abundance has affected everyone, and people of all ages, backgrounds, and occupations are equally unequipped to process all the information, products, and activities being pushed upon them today. You are living in a unique historical period in which people generally have more things and thoughts than ever before but are finally facing the limits to growth. You may want to simplify, streamline, get to the essence of what's important, and at the end of the day have more time and money and less stress and stuff. But how?

Let's tackle the problem at the root, by looking at the causes of clutter.

* **Information overload.** Knowledge is power, but information you don't need is clutter. Getting organized will help you filter information flow and turn the tide of this new age to your advantage at work and play.

* **The drive to buy.** My main message when it comes to managing the drive to buy is: Be very afraid. Salespeople are pros. Advertisers go to school, attend training sessions, and earn advanced degrees finding ways to sell you things without regard for your needs. Their sole purpose is to sap your bank account and fill your available space. Then, surprise! You don't end up with the more fulfilling lifestyle they promised. Your big reward is an empty savings account and an overstuffed house.

* **Sale: Your favorite four-letter word.** Suddenly, shopping is not a matter of looking for what you came for but of choosing from what the store has put on sale. You're no longer matching a solution to a need. As you organize yourself and your home, you'll find it easier to put up a stop sign between you and the sale sign. You'll think of your nice neat closet . . . your nice full wallet . . . and you'll just say no.

* **Freebies.** Even more appealing than a sale to your bargain-hunting soul is that other four-letter word: *free*. Free lunch, free toothbrush, free trip for two to Bermuda — this single syllable is a siren call to all acquirers. But free offers usually have a price. Either the item comes attached to something else that you have to buy and may not want, or you have to buy more later, or you have to spend time filling out rebate forms and matching them to receipts and getting them in the mail. Maybe you spend 15 minutes filling out a $1 rebate. Isn't your time worth more than $4 an hour? Add in the cost of the stamp and the envelope, and you're really in the hole.

* **Warning: This car stops at garage sales.** Many cars have such a bumper sticker. If you're starting to see your house fill up with all the things you buy at garage sales, take a look at what's happening: Everyone else is putting out their clutter, and you're taking it home and making it yours. How can you recover from this organizing error? Turn around and have your own garage sale. What came in the front door goes out the garage door. (In the future, of course, you want to try not to let clutter in any door at all.) For ideas on having your own garage sale, see the Top Ten Lists at the end of this book.

❋ **Gifts that keep on taking.** A gift, almost by definition, is something you didn't choose — so you may or may not want it. But a gift is also a token of affection or esteem, so you have to keep it, right? The important thing to remember about gifts is that they're meant to make you happy. Clutter doesn't do that. Clutter messes up your life. So observe the true spirit of giving by returning to the store gifts you don't want, exchanging them for something you can use, or putting the refund money in the kids' college fund.

❋ **Saving for later.** Did your parents teach you to save for a rainy day? Go have a garage sale, get rid of all the junk, and put the cash in the bank for the day you lose your job, leave your relationship, or make another major life change. Clothes you can't or don't wear anymore, old appliances and dinner plates, outdated files and papers, and extra boxes of staples simply aren't going to make the difference on that rainy day. Though someday may always seem just around the corner, the chapters that follow will help you make more of today by clearing away the clutter you're saving for later. Focusing on the present can yield many future benefits.

❋ **Souvenirs and mementos.** Souvenirs are another form of saving for later, trying to capture a moment in a thing. When travel becomes a quest to acquire objects to remember you were there instead of devoting yourself to being there, you're cheating yourself now and cluttering up your later.

Why get organized? To collect the payoff of putting everything in its place: More time and less stress. Cash in your pocket and peace of mind. Peak productivity, better health, and more rewarding relationships.

Flip through the pages of this book to see how you can put organization to work for you — from planning a meal to pulling off a strategic project, from beautifying your home to cleaning up your computer. Get organized so you can make more of your life while working less, and let these proven systems take care of the rest.

Maintaining Organization

Many people are hesitant to put the effort into getting organized because they doubt they can maintain an organized state of affairs. Like going on a diet, why bother if the excess pounds or clutter are just going to come back?

The beauty of getting organized is that it does retrain your mind, and no biochemical cues are trying to confuse the message. In fact, organization is one of those self-reinforcing pleasures in which a mind and body, grateful for the reduced stress and strain, are eager to explore more. Enter maintenance.

Part 1: Getting Started

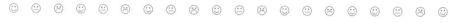

If you follow the systems described in this book, you may only need to have a major organizing session once a year or less to clean up any given area. A few basic tactics common to all these systems make maintenance easy. Here they are, for the benefit of your newly organizing mind:

❋ **Right now.** Clean up clutter as soon as you create it.

❋ **Every day.** Spend 15 minutes at the end of each day putting things away so tomorrow is a brand-new start.

❋ **The one-year rule.** Every time you come across an object or piece of paper, ask yourself if you've used it in the past year. If the answer is no, chances are the item can go.

❋ **Plan and schedule.** If a major organizing job arises, don't sit around waiting to have the time to take on a grand action. Break it down into chunks today and write each upcoming task on your calendar.

❋ **Set routines.** Establish patterns, from the annual purging of everyone's closets before buying new school clothes to repaving the blacktop driveway to weekly grocery shopping, laundry, or housecleaning on the same day each week, and so on. Clean out the china cabinet and the garage each spring and fall. Write the car's oil changes on your calendar. Straighten up the house the day before its weekly cleaning. Purge a few files every day. The more routines you can set, the faster and smoother things can go and the stronger your organizational systems can be.

❋ **Share.** Remember that maintenance isn't your job alone. Set up systems to share with your family.

The seeds are planted in your mind. All you need to do is fertilize them with all the information herein, and then watch your organized self blossom forth.

Chapter 2

Preparing to Succeed: Tools, Supplies, Systems

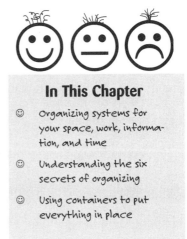

Getting organized is a systematic process, so it makes sense that there are some systems and supplies that go into making it work. On this subject, there is good news and good news. First, the right resources, from pullout drawers for your desktop to a calendar/planner matched to your scheduling needs, can make organizing far easier than you may have thought. Second, when you assemble the right resources to get organized, you don't need many. Some key containers and time-management tools, a small selection of information-management supplies, and six simple organizing procedures you can easily carry in your head to handle any organizing question are the sum total of what you need to change your life for the better.

Paper Clips, File Folders, Binders: What's It All About?

Stocking your desk and office right is half the fight for productive and efficient work. In Chapter 10, you can find out how to divide and organize your desktop and drawers into task-driven *centers,* and how to choose and use office supplies.

An organized approach to office supplies saves time and money and makes every job easier, so no matter what your position or post, take the time to simplify and supplement your supplies as Chapter 10 describes.

☺ ☹ ☺ ☺ ☺ ☺ ☺ ☺ ☺ ☺ ☺ ☺ ☺ ☺ ☺ ☺ ☺ ☺ ☺ ☺ ☺

Whether you're organizing at home or the office, you probably have plenty of paper and electronic information to deal with. The right tools can keep information in its place, which is right at your fingertips.

At work and home, all active papers are best kept in file folders inside hanging files. Loose files fall over, and loose papers do not make the organizing grade. The same goes for loose computer files running around your hard drive with no rhyme or reason. Inactive papers and electronic files need a space of their own, located outside your prime productive area and with the same system for easy additions and retrievals.

The basic tools for any paper filing system include:

❀ Drawers or containers

❀ Hanging files

❀ Hanging-file tabs

❀ File folders

❀ File-folder labels

Add in binders and perhaps a few file pockets and wallets, as well as a color-coding system for your tabs and labels, and there's no piece of paper you can't tame. Discover everything you need to know about the ABCs of filing for office or home in Chapter 10.

Organizers and Planners: Lists to Live By

Organized people don't trust their memory — they trust their lists. Two lists can manage your time, plain and simple. You start with a Master List, which, just as it sounds, covers everything in your life — sort of an ongoing download from your mind. The Master List flows to your To Do List, the tool for scheduling your day, meeting your deadlines, and achieving your goals.

After you have your lists in place, filling in your planner and putting it to work is as easy as pie. Chapter 15 explores all your organizer options — electronic, paper, or both; daily, weekly, or monthly; large or small; filled with this feature or that. You'll even find out what color to write which engagements in. If you haven't tapped the full power of a planner before, getting organized on this front can fill a big gap in your potential.

When you go shopping for your organizer, here are a few formats and names you may see:

❀ **Paper and paper-to-electronic systems:** At a Glance, DayTimers, Day Runners, Filofax, Franklin Covey. Old-fashioned paper has several advantages even in the twenty-first century: easy access, portability, and the ability to flip quickly and scan your schedule at a glance.

* **Electronic systems:** *PDAs*, or Personal Digital Assistants (like the Palm Pilot, Casio iPAQ, Hewlett Packard Jornada, HandSpring Visor, and Sony Clie) and various computer programs such as Microsoft Outlook. With the power to carry and categorize vast amounts of information, many electronic organizers also offer access to the Internet and e-mail via your Internet connection for computer programs, and through a wireless connection for portable devices.

* **Internet-based systems:** If you have a computer, but you don't yet have an electronic organizer, you can get started with electronic planning using a free Internet calendar system, like Yahoo. Signing up is easy, and if you choose to get a PDA or use a system like Outlook later, you can *sync* (or synchronize) your appointments, events, and special dates any time. If you're more the paper-planner type, you can print out your day's, week's or month's events with the touch of a button.

You can spend anything from less than $10 to several hundred on an organizer, depending upon whether you choose paper or electronic and how many features and add-ons you want. The information in Chapter 15 will help you reach the right cost-benefit ratio when it's time to shop for your planner.

Putting Things in Their Place: Containers

Every time you set out to organize a space, you need containers to clean out the deadwood and create homes for the survivors. Whether you're working in the garage or getting your office into shape, the following tools and techniques can help put everything into place.

No-strain containers: Types, shapes, and sizes

Containers can organize things by like type, such as trays for cosmetics or pens and pencils or dividers for desk or underwear drawers. They can keep food fresh, as a sealed canister does your pasta or pet food. Containers can facilitate cleanup — for instance, put preschoolers' toys in big open baskets that children can access easily. From the kitchen to the office, the boardroom to the bath, containers are your organizing friends.

 Whenever you aim to contain, measure the item(s) and storage space first, and then search the house or hit the store for what you need.

Containing options include:

* Cabinets

* Shelves

☺ ☻ ☹ ☺ ☻ ☹ ☺ ☻ ☹ ☺ ☻ ☹ ☺ ☻ ☹ ☺ ☺ ☻ ☹ ☺

❀ Drawers and drawer dividers

❀ Bookcases and bookends

❀ Magazine racks

❀ File drawers and boxes

❀ Baskets, boxes, and a variety of closed containers

❀ Tiered and stacking racks

Each class of container comes in a range of materials, shapes, and sizes. Matching these characteristics to your containing criteria is your goal — so isn't it great that manufacturers have come out with just about every container you could ever need?

Selecting the material

In selecting material, consider the container's weight, durability, safety, and looks, and whether you can lift or carry it easily. In general, plastic is lightest, lasts long, and doesn't break. However, plastic is often not as scenic as glass or a pretty basket. You probably don't want plastic in your living room, but boy, is it great in the kitchen, inside cupboards, and for storage areas.

Doing geometry: Shape and size

Round containers waste space. Want to picture why? Square off a round container in your mind's eye and you can see the corners that you're losing. Or put several round containers together and look at all the empty space in between. Whenever you can, choose squares or rectangles for your containers to avoid this geometric rip-off. Yes, you'll need some round bowls, and a big round basket works well for balls, but otherwise stick to the squares.

When you have the basic geometry down, match the shape and size of containers to what you're storing there. Allow enough space to group things by like type, but not so much that things get lost or jumbled within the container or you're left with a lot of room to spare.

Also ask yourself whether you need a lid on this container. Does it need a tight seal or stackable surface? Some containers, such as Tupperware's Modular Mates, stack easily on top of each other, which can make good use of vertical space.

Identifying with labels

A label can save loads of time by identifying a container's contents with a quick look. Best for things you're storing out of sight, container labels add information to your organization. Here are a few tips:

❀ Be sure to use a washable label if you may be cleaning the container in question (for instance, the one you store your flour in).

✤ Clear labels are hard to see on clear containers. If you use a clear, washable label on a clear container, place the label low so that the contents behind it can serve as a background.

✤ Use colored labels to code containers by type. Maybe all your baking supplies are in containers with blue labels (*b* is for blue and for baking), while pasta and grains are labeled with green (*g* for green and grains).

Just as firefighters talk about containing fires, use containers to contain clutter and spend less time putting out organizational fires. Containers provide a place for every important item in your life.

The Three Ds: Using containers as clutter busters

What are the Three Ds? Three containers that you use anytime you tackle a space to *distribute, donate,* or *dump* the stuff you find there. Here's how the Three Ds can ease the flow of things and keep you clutter-free.

Distribute box

Have you ever noticed how things tend to end up where they don't belong? To bring them on home, take a container and label it "Distribute." When you find a cereal bowl in the bedroom, don't rush downstairs to take it to the kitchen, and then go back up to collect the dirty clothes and run them down to the laundry room, followed by a stop in the front hall to grab the suntan lotion you had out for yesterday's tennis game and return it to the upstairs linen closet, and so on and so on until you're utterly exhausted. Five minutes of simple cleanup can wipe you out for the day unless you centralize operations with a distribute box.

A Halfway House: A container for the undecided

You may have a hard time parting with things. (If you didn't, you wouldn't need to read this book.) Sometimes, though, all you really need is time. Let time heal the pain of parting by putting the items you can't quite say goodbye to into a box. Mark it with "Halfway House" and the date. If a year rolls by and you haven't gone into the box for something you wanted, then give it away, unopened. This is important. If you open the box, you're likely to pull something back out into your home. So don't. If you really want something from your Halfway House during the cooling off period, go get it. Then close up the box and proceed to give the remaining contents away if you don't pull them out within a year.

Any time you need to leave the room to put something away, don't. Put it in the distribute box instead, and then carry it along to the next stop, just like riders on the bus waiting to exit until they reach home.

Donate box

Maybe the item is not out of place but it no longer has a place in your life. When that's the case, consider donating. Anything useable but no longer useful to you goes in the donate box, which sits there waiting to go to your sister, neighbor, or favorite charity for a tax write-off. For instance, if you have three sizes of clothes in your closet, you obviously aren't wearing two of them, so donate those. You probably don't want to go back to the larger size, and when you reach the smaller one, you'll deserve a treat of some new clothes in today's styles. The same goes for appliances, equipment (donate or sell computer stuff the second it gets disconnected from your system; those things aren't getting any younger), dishes, furniture — you name it. Letting things move on to people who can use them makes the world a better place, and your donate box can help.

Dump box

Then there are things that nobody wants or needs. You can designate a box, trash can, or big garbage bag for things you choose to dump as you unclutter. The trick is to keep it close at hand as you work and put anything you want to discard directly into the garbage.

The Six Organizing Secrets

Five of the organizing secrets are *acronyms,* words in which each letter stands for a step of the process to make each one easy to remember. Simply remembering the six organizing secrets and putting the secrets to work can help train your organizing mind.

Designing any space with a layout

When you start out to tackle a space, the ideal first question takes in the big picture: "Where do things *go?*" Is that the best arrangement for the desk and filing cabinets? Can you open up more space by moving the bed? What's the most efficient use of the room's wall space? To answer the big-picture question, think like an architect.

Even if you've never sat down at a drafting table, you can lay out any space by drawing, cutting, and playing. Specific goals and considerations for rooms in the home and office are covered in their individual chapters. For now, take a moment to review the basics of how easy it is to make like an architect and create your own blueprint for high-performance rooms. Just follow these simple steps:

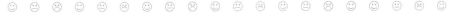

1 **Draw the basic blueprint.**

First, get out a tape measure and measure the dimensions of the space you want to organize, including the width of each wall, window, door, and closet, as well as the height underneath windows. Jot down each measurement as you go.

Now swap your tape measure for a ruler and draw your room to scale on a blank piece of paper, using 1 inch to represent 1 foot. Tape two sheets of paper together if you need to. After sketching the basic outline, mark the windows, including a note about the wall clearance underneath, the closets, and the doors.

2 **Create cutouts.**

Now think about what furniture and equipment you want in the room — including what's there now, new items as recommended in the chapters, or something that's been on your wish list. Measure these items if you already have them or estimate their dimension if not. Next, take some colored paper and cut out a rectangle, square, or circle to represent each piece, again using 1 inch to represent 1 foot as your scale. A typical desk is about 6 feet long and 3 feet wide, so that becomes a 6-x-3-inch rectangular cutout.

Continue until you cover all the furniture and equipment you'd like to include in your layout. Be sure to write what each cutout represents on the front so you don't lose track.

3 **Play with your layout.**

Finally, put glue (or sticky tack) that allows you to reposition your layout on the backs of the cutouts so you can move them around on your blueprint but not lose their place, and play with your layout. Remember to use the space under windows for smaller pieces — a desk or two-drawer file cabinet in an office, or a dresser or short bookcase in the home. Also keep in mind that doors need room to open and close, so don't put the fax machine in the door's path.

Keep playing until you come up with one or more layouts you like. You may discover a whole new look for your room, or that there's not enough space for the bed and bureau to share a wall, all without lifting a finger or straining your back. Not bad for your first organizing secret.

Saving or tossing

How do you decide what to keep and what's a waste of space and time — not to mention energy and money? Simply ask the five W-A-S-T-E questions, and you're well on your way to an informed keep-or-toss decision. As you work through the questions, think like a judge, considering past precedent, future ramifications, and sometimes-subjective differences between right and wrong:

☺ ☻ ☹ ☺ ☻ ☹ ☺ ☻ ☹ ☺ ☻ ☹ ☺ ☻ ☹ ☺ ☺ ☻ ☹ ☺

❋ **Worthwhile:** Do you truly like the dress or shirt in question? Is that article actually important to your job? Does the fax cover sheet contain any information you need to know? If the item isn't worthwhile, toss it out now. If it is, move on to the next four bullets.

❋ **Again:** Will you really use this thing again, or is it just going to sit in a kitchen cupboard or take up space in your files? This item could also be rephrased as, "Use it or lose it." If you don't foresee needing something in the next year or you haven't used it in the last one, clear it out. Maybe you used your waffle iron weekly for a while but you haven't touched it in months because you broke up with the boyfriend you cooked them for or got tired of cleaning out the grooves. It was once worthwhile, but now, goodbye!

❋ **Somewhere else:** Ask yourself, "Can I easily find this somewhere else?" If you have to make waffles for a special brunch, can you borrow a waffle iron from a neighbor? Can you find a memo in your assistant's files or in another department, or get the details by making a quick phone call? Can you hit the Internet, the library, or the local discount store if the need for this item or info should arise in the future? A good way to avoid this sort of redundancy is to say, "Out with the old and in with the new."

❋ **Toss:** Many things have ways of slipping and sliding by the first three questions, so here's the acid test: Will anything happen if you toss it? If not, go ahead, unless it must be retained for legal reasons. (Chapter 14 gives you guidelines for retaining information.) This question often ends up taking people on a sentimental journey. Maybe something passed the first three questions because it had sentimental value, but the world wouldn't stop turning if that item were tossed. This question is the toughest to judge because it can't be measured by anyone but you. The sentimental value of things generally accrues from the people who gave them to you, whether a family elder, a good friend or lover, or — here's a hot button — a child.

❋ **Entire:** Do you need the entire thing? The whole magazine, document, or draft? Every coordinate of the outfit, even if you only ever wear the pants? The complete catalog, when you only intend to order from one page? If not, keep what you need and toss the excess.

Everything in its P-L-A-C-E: Organizing space

Are you looking for a way to clear an area of clutter, organize items for easy access and neat appearance, and fine-tune the results to your needs. P-L-A-C-E is the way to organize space and put everything in its place. What could be easier to remember?

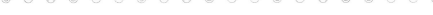

You can clean up any area in the world with the following five steps:

❋ **Purge:** First, break out the Three Ds and the five W-A-S-T-E questions and clear your space of clutter by dumping, donating, or distributing everything you no longer need (see the preceding sections). Whether you toss out the dried-up glue sticks in your desk drawer, discard outgrown toys in the playroom, or clean the hall closet of unmatched gloves and ratty old sweatshirts, purging can empower all your organizing efforts.

❋ **Like with like:** The second step in putting things into place is to organize like things together. Not only does grouping help you know where to look, whether you're searching for a file or a first-aid lotion, but placing similar items together also often creates what I call *centers*, one-stop spots with everything you need to complete a task.

❋ **Access:** After you have things grouped, placement is the next priority — and here, think easy access. Where do you usually use these items? Put them there. Pots and pans should be near the stove and file cabinets close to your desk. How close is close? Literally at your fingertips.

❋ **Contain:** Containers do double-duty from an organizing perspective: They keep like things together and move things out of sight to clear the landscape and your mind. The more you contain, the better you may feel, and you can find an abundance of practical ideas, complete with pictures and illustrations, in the coming chapters.

❋ **Evaluate:** After you complete the first four steps of P-L-A-C-E, Evaluate: Does it work? Organization is an ongoing process, and organizing can often be improved upon as your needs change or you sharpen your skills. You'll find evaluation questions throughout these chapters to help you size up the success of each project as you finish it and in the future.

When you evaluate and adjust over time, your organization systems become self-maintaining. Some good occasions to assess your systems include changing jobs, starting college, getting your first apartment, getting married, getting divorced, and moving.

Clearing your desktop with R-E-M-O-V-E

You may be reading this book because you can't see the surface of your desk and have no idea how to fix the situation short of a snowplow. That's why R-E-M-O-V-E, six steps to clear off even the most snowed-under desktop and set a desk up for success, is the key. You'll find more details on this in Chapter 10, but here's a quick preview to get you thinking:

- **Reduce distractions:** Is your desk covered with pictures, knick-knacks, or this morning's mail? These may be distracting you and reducing productivity. The reduce principle helps you to identify distractions and get them off your desk.

- **Everyday use:** Only things that you use every day may stay on top of your desk. Don't worry; you'll find homes for everything else you need.

- **Move to the preferred side:** You use one hand for most daily operations, and your desk can be arranged accordingly. Placing pens, pencils, and pads where you reach for them most gives you fingertip management and makes everything from writing notes to taking phone calls faster and easier. See Chapter 10 for the big exception to the preferred side rule. Can you guess?

- **Organize together:** Just as with P-L-A-C-E, organizing like things together on the desktop forms centers so you can find and use items easily.

- **View your time:** Everybody hates to be late, so give yourself a leg up by making time visual on your desk. An organizer and a clock are important desktop elements for keeping time in view.

- **Empty the center:** Finally, chanting the mantra that "The desk is a place to do work," clear off a space in the center of the station so that you can work on the project at hand. Behold, a long-lost surface — your desk!

Responding to your mail with R-A-P-I-D

Even before e-mail came on the scene, mail overload had slowed many people down to a snail's pace, so this system is designed to help you pick up speed with a R-A-P-I-D sort that doesn't even require opening an envelope. Five sort categories help you bring order to incoming mail and get it opened and filed in a flash. Here they are:

- **Read:** Anything that you need to read — later, please — goes in this stack. You may often find *to read* items at the bottom of the mail pile because they're big ol' magazines and newsletters.

- **Attend:** Notices and invitations for seminars, workshops, meetings, performances, parties, and so forth go in the *to attend* stack.

- **Pay:** If somebody wants your money, *to pay* is the pile to put the item in. Window envelopes are an easy cue. If it looks like one more credit card offer you don't want, just rip right through the envelope to protect your identity and toss, all without taking the time to open it. Time is money, and all these folks are already after yours.

❀ **Important:** Presume important until proven innocent, and put all unknown incoming mail into this stack.

❀ **Dump:** If you know at a glance that you won't read or need it, do *not* break the seal on the envelope. *Do* dump that piece of mail in the nearest available trash can.

Chapter 14 walks you through R-A-P-I-D in detail and tells you what to do with mail after you open the envelope.

Maximizing your time with P-L-A-N

The most important thing you can plan is your time, that precious and irreplaceable commodity. Yes, there's more to it than simply marking dates in your calendar, but planning time doesn't have to be hard. All you need are four steps formulated to take you to your goals, large or small. Put time on your side and achieve your peak potential with the power of P-L-A-N:

❀ **Prepare:** The step you all too often skip in dividing up your time on Earth is defining missions and setting goals. The result can be that instead of pursuing what you want and need, you simply do whatever presents itself to you.

❀ **Lists you can live by:** Out of your goals flow things to do, and the Master and To Do lists keep track of all these tasks over the short and long term so you can do more and stress less. When you find out how to use these lists along with your daily planner, you need never let a small detail or top priority slip again.

❀ **Act with rhythms and routines:** Time has rhythms, like the ticking of the clock, the beating of your heart, and the biochemical changes your body and brain go through every day. When you discover how to act with your personal rhythms and establish timesaving routines, you may find more minutes in the day and reap better results from all your efforts. From sleeping to peaking to pacing, acting with rhythms and routines helps you go with the flow.

❀ **Notice and reward your accomplishments:** Here comes the fun part: Whenever you accomplish a goal, you earn yourself a reward, and the P-L-A-N system makes sure you get one by building a prize right into the time-management process. When you notice and reward your accomplishments, you create an even stronger incentive to reach your goal the next time around. Pretty soon you have a positive feedback loop that can spiral you right to the moon.

Part 1: Getting Started

☺ ☻ ☹ ☺ ☻ ☹ ☺ ☻ ☹ ☺ ☻ ☹ ☺ ☻ ☹ ☺ ☺ ☻ ☹ ☺

Part 2

Organizing Your Primary Living Spaces

This part applies the basic organizing systems to the specific rooms of your home. Whether you want to clear off your counters; create a soothing, relaxing master suite; or rearrange your home office, there's something for everyone in this part. Look for ways to create a multi-tasking family room in Chapter 4. Find great ideas for setting up separate centers in your playroom in Chapter 5. And don't miss back-saving kitchen storage tips in Chapter 3. Skip around, or read it straight through. You're bound to pick up helpful tips in each and every chapter.

Chapter 3

Having a Clutter-Free Kitchen

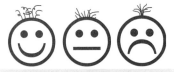

Organizing the kitchen can seem like a big job, so don't try to tackle the task all at once. Choose a single section, such as straightening up the pantry or arranging pots and pans, to get started.

Making a P-L-A-C-E for Everything

Whether you work your way straight through this chapter or skip around from one section to another, your successes can inspire you to continue until everything is in its P-L-A-C-E — the word that summarizes the five steps to cleaning up your kitchen as follows:

❀ **Purge:** Toss out broken or worn items, from appliances you haven't fixed to dull kitchen knives that you don't plan to sharpen. The same goes for outgrown kids' dishes and cleaning supplies you tried but didn't like. In the pantry, fridge, and freezer, anything old or unidentifiable goes in the garbage. Say goodbye to expired coupons and untried or unsuccessful recipes. Do you have appliances, dishes, or pans that you don't use but someone else could? Donate!

❀ **Like with like:** Group items of similar type together, including dishes, utensils, pots and pans, appliances, and cleaning supplies. Arrange pantry, refrigerator, and freezer shelves like supermarket sections.

☺ ☹ ☺ ☺ ☺ ☺ ☺ ☺ ☺ ☺ ☺ ☹ ☺ ☺ ☺ ☺ ☺ ☺ ☹ ☺

❀ **Access:** Place appliances, dishes, pots and pans, and utensils closest to their most frequent use, creating one-stop centers to make coffee, cook at the stove, serve meals, package leftovers, and wash dishes. Heavier items can go on lower shelves, while lighter things can be kept in cupboards above the countertop. Move seldom-used items to out-of-the-way cabinets or their deepest corners. Sink stuff that you don't use every day can be stored in the cabinet below.

❀ **Contain:** Move non-everyday items (appliances, cutting boards, knives) off countertops and into cabinets and drawers. Add dividers to drawers to contain their contents by type. Transfer grain products from boxes and bags to sealed plastic or glass containers. Organize recipes and restaurant reviews into binders and coupons into a 4-x-6-inch file box.

❀ **Evaluate:** Do you have enough counter space to prep foods, accommodate dirty dishes, and serve meals with ease? Can you make coffee, clean and chop vegetables and get the trimmings into the garbage or disposal, and wash dishes from start to finish — each without taking more than a step? Are you comfortable cooking, eating, and hanging out in the kitchen?

Clearing Off Your Countertops

Surfaces you can see are a good place to start organizing your kitchen, because visible areas have both aesthetic and practical importance. Clear counters provide space to work and promote peace of mind while you cook, as well as looking much nicer than the appliance junkyard that clutters many a kitchen.

Identifying countertop criteria

Access is the key criterion to apply when clearing off countertops. Three cardinal questions can qualify an item, be it an appliance or a knife block, for residence on your counter. Ask yourself:

❀ **Do you use it every day?** If the answer is yes, that's a countertop contender. Qualifying examples may include the coffeemaker, toaster, microwave, can opener, and knife set.

❀ **Is a convenient under-the-counter version available?** Kitchen basics from paper-towel holders to clock/radios to can openers and even toasters are now made to mount under counters and free up valuable space.

❀ **Can the item fit into an easy-access cabinet near where you use it?** If the answer is yes, and this is not an everyday item, you've just found its new home. *Exception:* Take into account the heaviness of the item and the height of the cupboard. You may not mind reaching overhead for a coffee grinder, but wrestling a Mixmaster out of a high or low cabinet is asking for trouble.

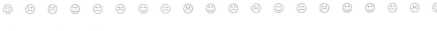
Arranging the countertop

After passing countertop clearance, an item needs a location. As with any prime real estate, carefully consider the space on your counter, including where an item is most commonly and conveniently accessed. The key to a cool kitchen is fingertip management, in which you arrange everything from soap to soup bowls according to a *work center* concept of accomplishing basic tasks without taking a step. Apply the fingertip management concept to everything you do to cook, serve, clean up, pack lunches, and unpack groceries. Here are some principles for easy-access counters:

❁ Electrical appliances need to go near an outlet the cord can reach.

❁ Put the toaster near the plate cupboard for easy early-morning serving.

❁ To create a coffee center, situate the coffeemaker somewhere near the sink so you can fill and empty the pot in the same spot. Store the coffee, filters, mugs, sugar bowl, and creamer in a cupboard overhead. For you purists who grind your own, put the grinder and beans here, too.

❁ A can opener located near the sink makes draining off liquid and wiping up spills easy.

❁ The microwave should be in easy reach — lifting down hot dishes is a home safety hazard — and near a heatproof surface (tile counter, stovetop, or wooden board).

❁ The food processor, blender, and juicer are swing items. Store them in a cupboard if they're rarely turned on; otherwise, find a spot on the counter somewhere near the refrigerator, if possible, so ingredients are within close reach.

Clearing off your countertops can have an immediate enlightening effect that inspires the rest of your kitchen makeover. With all this wide-open space, you can shift your focus to the food you're preparing and the pleasure of the people around you.

Simplifying Your Sink

The phrase *and the kitchen sink* was coined to describe anything and everything thrown together any which way. If your kitchen sink is in such a state of chaos, simplify. Stand at your sink and ask yourself: What do I do where? Answering that question can help you create your sink centers.

Creating the dishwashing center

If you have a two-sided sink, in one side you probably wash the dishes, and in the other side you probably scrape (if the sink has a garbage disposal) or rinse. Start by putting your soap, sponge, scrubber, and brush on the washing side.

☺ ☻ ☹ ☺ ☻ ☹ ☺ ☻ ☹ ☺ ☻ ☹ ☺ ☻ ☹ ☺ ☺ ☻ ☹ ☺

Try these ideas for completing your dishwashing makeover:

✿ If your sink boasts a built-in pump for dish soap, use it. This gets the bottle out of the way and provides easier, neater dispensing.

✿ As an alternative, try an attractive pump bottle for the dish soap, one purchased for the purpose or a recycled hand-soap bottle (in colors that match your kitchen). To prevent clogging, rinse the spout after use.

✿ Go tubular with a *single soap-sponge unit,* a sponge attached to a tube that you fill with soap, which means your sponge is always soaped up and ready to go. The downside is that the device can make a soapy mess while lying around, and the tube requires refilling more often than a soap bottle does.

✿ Try a nifty little sponge basket with two suction cups on the back that gloms onto the wall inside the sink and keeps two or more sponges — maybe a soft one for wiping counters and a nylon rib sponge for scrubbing pans — virtually out of sight.

✿ Presoaped pot scrubbers can go into a raised soap dish with a drain to keep them out of rust-making, soap-leaching water.

✿ Install a tilt-down panel/drawer at the front of the sink — just the spot for your sponges.

Under the sink: Cleaning and supply center

The term *sinkhole* may come to mind when you consider that dark place down under. Rediscover this treasure trove of usable space by setting it up as a cleaning and supply center. Placement is everything under the sink, and if yours is a tangled thicket, think access in front-to-back rows. The front row includes anything you use every day or so — dishwasher soap, kitchen cleanser, and rubber gloves. The next row is for less-frequently used items such as other cleansers and cleaning supplies, soap refills, and laundry detergent (if you don't have a laundry room). In the back, put your spare paper towels and sponges. Within each layer, keep like things together, using the left and right sides as natural subdivisions — for instance, paper towels go on the left, cleansers on the right. Don't forget to use vertical space by stacking when you can.

Classifying Your Cabinets and Drawers

Cabinets and drawers can attract clutter and make clatter. Nevertheless, properly classified, the secret space behind closed doors can be a cook's best friend.

Pots, pans, dishes, casseroles, and mixing bowls are usually best stored in stacks. Though retrieving an item at the bottom of a pile can be a major weight-lifting chore, so much space is saved that I recommend accepting stacks as a fact of life. Use racks with as many tiers as your shelf can accommodate to create stacks on top of stacks, making item removal and return much easier. Try the ones that expand to the height of your shelf for maximum stacking.

Dishes: Serving center

Decide where to put dishes depending upon where and how often you access them. The closer you keep frequently used dishes to the dishwasher and/or dish drainer, the quicker you get them put away. On the other end of the equation, you're well served to keep dishes close to where you usually use them — the stove for dinner plates, refrigerator for sandwich plates, and so on. Look for the best tradeoff between serving and stowing locations.

There are matters of altitude to consider, too. Save your lower cupboards for hefty pots and pans, and place dishes on shelves above the counter. Heavy dinner plates work well on the lowest shelf of an upper cabinet, with salad and sandwich plates and bowls just above.

 Make more out of a tall shelf with a three-tiered coated wire rack. Putting dinner plates on one tier, salad plates on another, and bowls on the third beats making one big stack and having to move the whole mountain every time you want something from the bottom.

Glasses, cups, and mugs: Beverage center

Put kid glasses and plastic cups at a kid-friendly height so you don't have to be bothered every time a child wants a drink. Mugs can go higher up, because (unless you're raising coffee hounds) kids only use them for the occasional hot chocolate.

Organize your glass cupboard by starting with the shortest glasses on one side and working your way to the tallest on the other, in columns of the same height or glass type. No more fumbling toward the back for the glass you want. Again, if your cupboard is tall, a coated wire rack can double your usable space. Make sure the clearance between shelves accommodates your tallest glasses.

Pots and pans: Cooking center

Though modern metals technology has taken us a long way from the days of 10-ton cast-iron skillets, pots and pans are still big and heavy. That's why you want to think *low* when you consider cabinet space for cooking vessels.

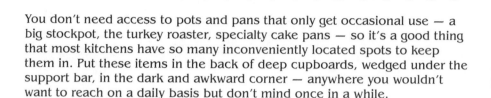
You don't need access to pots and pans that only get occasional use — a big stockpot, the turkey roaster, specialty cake pans — so it's a good thing that most kitchens have so many inconveniently located spots to keep them in. Put these items in the back of deep cupboards, wedged under the support bar, in the dark and awkward corner — anywhere you wouldn't want to reach on a daily basis but don't mind once in a while.

 Remembering what you've got stored in hard-to-reach cabinets can be hard. Give your brain a break by posting a list, like the one in Table 3-1, of contents on the inside of the cabinet door.

Table 3-1 Cabinet Contents

Pans in This Cabinet	On Which Shelf?
Extra-large roasting pan	Bottom
Bread machine	Bottom

After you divvy up the least-desirable space, put the rest of your pots and pans in the slots closest to their point of use. Skillets and saucepans can go in the bottom drawer of the stove, and baking sheets and cooling racks into a tall, narrow cabinet alongside. (If you don't have such a cabinet, get a set of dividers designed to stand baking sheets and racks on end.) Casseroles, baking dishes, mixing bowls, cutting boards, and cake and pie tins are conveniently stored under the food-prep counter.

To store lids space-efficiently, put one lid knob-side down inside of your stack of pans, and then layer on another lid knob-side up, like a sandwich.

 Square edges align and round ones don't, so the simple truth is that anything round wastes cabinet space. Choose square pans when you can.

☺ ☻ ☹ ☺ ☺ ☻ ☹ ☺ ☻ ☹ ☺ ☻ ☹ ☺ ☻ ☹ ☺ ☺ ☻ ☹ ☺

The Drawer Doctor Is In

Kitchen drawers can easily fall into disarray, with jumbled utensils and unsorted silverware getting in the way when you need a whisk to stir something on the stove or seek a salad fork. For drawers that do more, use the idea of work centers to create quick access to the tools for each type of task.

The five essential kitchen drawers are:

❁ **Tableware center:** Placed near the kitchen table, the tableware center drawer can include forks, spoons, table knives, and serving pieces.

❁ **Baking and prep utensil center:** Located near the counter and cutting board, the baking and prep utensil center should include measuring cups and spoons, mixing spoons, rubber scrapers, whisks, rolling pin, beaters, hand can opener, vegetable peeler, apple corer, garlic press, zester, egg separator, grater, food-processor discs, strainer, and kitchen shears.

❁ **Cooking utensil center:** Near the stove is the spot for the cooking utensil center, including spatulas, tongs, meat fork, ladle, slotted spoon, thermometers, potato masher, baster, and gravy separator. Utensils can stay cleaner inside a drawer — but if you simply don't have room, use a utensil stand on the counter by the stove instead.

❁ **Linen center:** Designate a drawer near the stove for potholders, mitts, kitchen towels, and cloths. No linen drawer? Hang your dishtowel on the oven bar and potholders from hooks on a wall above or near the stove. Keep extras in a pantry or cabinet shelf.

❁ **Office supply center:** Keep this area stocked with a freezer marker, masking and transparent tape, pens and pencils, scissors, ruler, and a stapler.

If you have a few more kitchen drawers

If you're blessed with a decadence of drawers and have more to spare, here are some other ideas:

❁ **Knife center:** Chopping, slicing, paring, and steak knives can go here. *Warning:* If you have small children, skip the countertop knife block and keep everything sharp put away in a drawer instead. Safety locks can keep small ones out of dangerous places such as a drawer full of knives or a cupboard with household cleaners and chemicals.

❁ **Wrap center:** The basics for this center include aluminum foil, resealable plastic bags, plastic wrap, wax paper, storage bags, and twist ties.

❁ **Coupon, box top, and proof-of-purchase center:** Keep these items only if you redeem them regularly; otherwise, they count as clutter and should go. (Read on for hints on coping with coupons.)

❋ **Basic tool center:** You need handy access to a screwdriver, hammer, nails, and pliers. You can add tools to your office supply center if you don't have a separate drawer to dedicate. **Remember:** Move tools to a high cabinet if you have young children who may hurt themselves.

Divide, conquer, and contain

When you have the right things in the right drawers, divide and conquer. Free-form drawers waste time and try your patience as you sort through in search of what you need — so measure your drawers, take stock of the size of the various items in them, and hit the store in search of dividers. Look for sections tailored to the length and width of the various things you store: standard tableware, measuring cups and spoons, gadgets, long knives, cooking utensils. Take advantage of the opportunity to give the insides of your drawers a good wipe-down before installing your new dividers.

 Don't buy dividers with slots molded to specific shapes, such as spoons. They limit your flexibility and drawer capacity. Get ultra-organized with the new self-adhesive section dividers that allow you to design the space to meet your needs.

Sectioning Off Your Pantry

Think of every visit to the pantry like a trip to the supermarket: You're shopping for what you need right now. Stores help you find things by arranging shelves by like type and making all items easy to access. You can do it, too. To put your pantry in the pink, use these eight great pantry sections:

❋ **Baking:** Sugars, flour, oatmeal, cornmeal, mixes (cake, brownie, pancake, muffin), baking powder and soda, salt, extracts, oil, shortening, chips, chocolate, pie fillings

❋ **Cereal:** Hot and cold breakfast cereals

❋ **Pasta and grains:** Dried pasta, noodles, rice, rice mixes, other grains, potato mixes, bread crumbs, stuffing

❋ **Canned fruits and vegetables:** Fruits, vegetables, applesauce, tomatoes, tomato sauce and paste, beans

❋ **Canned soup, entrees, meat, and fish:** Soup, broth, pasta, chili, tuna, salmon, chicken

❋ **Condiments:** Mustard, ketchup, mayonnaise, salad dressings, vinegar, sauces (marinara, hot sauce, barbeque, steak, chili, cocktail, soy, Worcestershire, salsa, and so on), peanut butter, jam and jelly

❋ **Snacks:** Chips, crackers, pretzels, rice cakes, cookies, ice-cream cones

☺ ☺ ☹ ☺ ☺ ☹ ☺ ☺ ☺ ☹ ☺ ☺ ☹ ☺ ☺ ☺ ☹ ☺ ☺ ☺ ☹ ☺

* **Drinks:** Coffee, tea, iced tea, hot chocolate, powdered creamers, sweeteners, drink mixes, soda, canned drinks, juice boxes, bottled water

 I've seen too many pantry shelves succumb to the pressure of super-sized foods and cases of soda. Avoid shelf sag or even breakage by putting your heaviest items on the floor or near support bars, and splitting up cans and jars. For instance, put fruits and vegetables on one shelf, canned soups and pastas on another, and condiments on a third.

After sectioning off the pantry, arrange items on shelves for easy access with two principles: above-below and front-to-back.

* **Above-below:** First, group each of the eight pantry sections on vertically adjacent shelves. For instance, you may place flour and sugar on the shelf directly above boxed mixes, chocolate chips, and other baking needs. The two-shelf approach helps compact the space for each section and distribute weight more evenly.

* **Front-to-back:** Next, put the tallest items at the back of the shelf and the shortest in front. That means tall cake mixes line up against the back wall, while pudding, gelatin, shortening, and nuts go in front. You can also use step shelves to add different levels to your front-back arrangements, as you see in Figure 3-1.

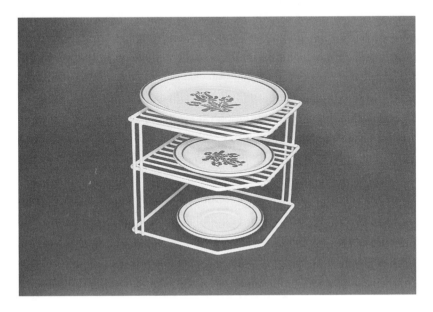

Figure 3-1: Use step shelves for plates, or to keep foods from playing hide-and-seek.

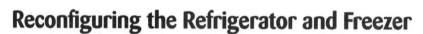

Reconfiguring the Refrigerator and Freezer

Like the pantry (but colder), the ideal refrigerator is arranged in supermarket-type sections with the taller items in back. You can adjust the height of most refrigerator shelves to accommodate your items without wasting space. But, you protest, I'd have to take everything out and start over! Yep. That's exactly what you need to do. (It's a great time to clean it out, too.)

The following steps can take you to a cleaner, more organized refrigerator:

1 Take it all out.

Pull up a trash bag and take everything out of the refrigerator, tossing fuzzy and old things as you go. Haven't used that mustard in a year? Goodbye! Give the whole thing a good swipe with a soapy sponge. Add an open box of baking soda to soak up refrigerator odors.

2 Start with the obvious.

Fruits and vegetables go in the bins (fruits on one side, vegetables on the other), cheese and deli items in the drawer if you have one, butter and cream cheese in the butter compartment, and eggs in the little indentations in the door.

3 Stock the door.

Fill the door shelves with smaller items grouped by like type — salad dressings, mustards, sauces, jams and jellies, and so on. Soda or milk up to quart size can go in taller door shelves; super-spacious doors can handle liters or even gallons. The door is also a convenient spot for a carton of half-and-half or creamer for splashing into coffee.

4 Work from the top.

The top shelf is the tallest, so this is the place for drinks. Adjust the shelf to suit your tallest pitcher or bottle. If you have split shelves, you can shorten up the other half and put your most frequently used items there (usually dairy).

5 Group foods by type and arrange them for easy access.

Look at what you have left to store and sort. Your sections may include cooked foods and leftovers; dairy products and eggs; meat, poultry, and seafood; and condiments. For each group, gauge the maximum height and adjust the shelf height accordingly.

Split shelf alert: A big sheet cake or lasagna waiting to hit the oven may not fit on a half-shelf. Get friendly with big foods by aligning at least one set of shelves to reach all the way across the fridge.

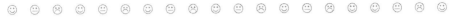

Now that you're cooled off, dig into the deep freeze. The same principles apply in the freezer as in the fridge: You want supermarket-like sections that make items easy to find by type. Achieve this by clearing out the contents, sorting items into sections, and selecting the freezer spots that afford best access to each group.

1 Toss the fossils.

Anything you don't recognize or remember or can't see through the frost gets tossed.

2 Section items off.

Seven good freezer sections include: meat, poultry, seafood, prepared entrees (store-bought or leftovers), sauces and side dishes, vegetables, juice concentrates, breads, and desserts.

3 Configure for access.

Freezer setups vary depending upon whether you have an above-fridge, below-fridge, side-by-side, or stand-alone unit. Whatever yours is, if you don't have enough shelves to make sense of your space, buy freestanding coated wire units with a few tiers. (Measure your freezer before shopping.) Next, arrange your food by section, with the items that you use most frequently closest at hand. Juice, breads, frozen vegetables, and desserts are often small enough to slip into door shelves.

Fast-Track Food Storage

You can get more out of your groceries when you store them right. Once you set up your system, unpacking groceries and putting away leftovers becomes a snap — and the contents of your kitchen stay organized and fresh.

Cool container solutions

Clear is the color of choice for food containers, whether plastic bags, glass canisters, or rectangular tubs. The instant visual ID a clear container offers can save you hours, maybe even years over the course of a lifetime. Colored labels and lids can provide aesthetic relief for your eye and a coding system for your mind.

Containers that go from the freezer to the microwave serve a dual purpose and save transfer time. Remember to go square for the best use of space. Stock a variety of sizes and stack the empties inside each other. If you're storing more containers than you're using, that's a tip to toss, as are any containers without a lid or vice versa. Set a quota. Keep, say, 10 large plastic containers and 13 small containers. When more come in, you need to pick your favorite containers and toss the others. Practice the "one in, one out" rule.

You can protect opened packages of grain products — including flour, oatmeal, cornmeal, rice, pasta, noodles, bread crumbs, stuffing mix, and dried beans — from insect invasion by storing them in containers with tightly sealing lids. Simply match the size of the container to the contents of your package, make the transfer, and then — don't forget this part or you may be sorry later — cut out any preparation instructions from the original package, wipe them clean, and put them right into the container for reference at cooking time. Tape prep instructions on the outside if you prefer, but keep in mind that removing the tape and paper when it's time to wash the container can be inconvenient.

Wrapping center

A wrap and packaging center can make quick work of leftovers, lunches, and food that you want to freeze in a one-stop spot. Find a drawer or cupboard shelf that can hold all your wraps — plastic wrap, aluminum foil, wax paper, sandwich bags, resealable bags, and lunch bags — and food containers in a variety of sizes. Containers can stack inside each other according to size.

After you get your wrap center set up with all your wrapping stuff, you're ready to prepare lunches, keep leftovers, and use your freezer to maximum efficiency. Here are some pro tips:

❀ Wrap foods in freezer paper, aluminum foil, or a double layer of plastic wrap, zip them into resealable plastic freezer bags, or slip them into plastic containers.

❀ Use a permanent marker or freezer pen to label and date everything as it goes in. Just a date will do on purchased items in their original wrapping. You can skip items you go through fast and use quickly.

❀ Color-code your labels or container lids according to the section they belong to or your own criteria. For instance, you can top beef-gravy containers with orange lids and turkey-gravy containers with beige. A quick-reference chart can help you decode your colors later; use the same ones all the time to remember better.

Mealtime or Hassletime: The Organized Meal Planner

The first step to master meal planning is to know what you eat. Take a minute to jot down what you ate for dinner each night for the past week. (If this is straining your brain, just keep a log for the next week or two.)

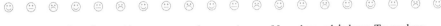

Now look for the pattern — maybe pasta on Monday; chicken Tuesday; meetings and school events on Wednesday (translation: leftovers or frozen entrees as everyone fends for themselves); tacos or wraps on Thursday; dinner out on Friday; Saturday, a slightly gourmet effort with fish or meat; and Sunday, takeout. Looks like you need to plan and shop for four nights. Not so hard, right (especially when you consider that most weeks run pretty much the same)?

Writing your master menu and grocery shopping list

Write up your typical week of meals, throwing in the lunches and break-fasts eaten at home. Add in any missing favorite and/or frequent meals. This is your master menu list.

Now use your menu list to create a master shopping list. Remember to account for fruits and veggies, side dishes, snacks, desserts, drinks, and school lunches. Organize your list by supermarket section, and then type it up and make a bunch of copies or enter it on your computer.

Keep your master lists on the bulletin board or in the office-supply drawer in the kitchen. Use the menu list to choose the next day's dinner before going to bed each night. Pull out a fresh copy of the shopping list each week and use a highlighter to indicate what you need. Add items to your current shopping list when they're halfway down. Stock a backup of any-thing you go through fast. Do you live in snow, earthquake, hurricane, tor-nado, or flood country? Keep some nonperishable items on hand for an emergency. If you live alone, you can stock some soups and canned foods for days that you're sick and can't go to the store.

Is making a master shopping list more than you can manage? There are two other solutions for you:

* **Keep a wipe-off board on the refrigerator door to write down things you need as you think of them during the week.** Let kids add their requests. On shopping day, jot down on a piece of paper all the items on the board. Look through your pantry and fridge and add whatever's running low as well as needs for the week's meals.

* **Use a magnetic shopping list with pieces to slide over the items you want to buy.** This method isn't as customized as a wipe-off board, but it's better than going without a list.

 Cooking in bulk truly saves time — and often money, because you can buy ingredients in value packs, and a well-stocked freezer or fridge can forestall many a stop at a restaurant or take-out place. Roasts, soups, stews, and casseroles are all great candidates for cooking ahead. So break out the big pots and leverage economy of scale. Remember to package the fruits of your labor in serving sizes right for one meal.

Shop like you mean it

An organized kitchen begins in the supermarket. If, like most people, you usually hit the store with frayed nerves and a scattered mind and come home with a predictably mixed bags of goods, try these shopping strategies to procure like a pro:

❀ **Shop at the right store.** Keep a separate list for bulk purchases — paper goods, cleaning supplies, soda, liquor, and nonperishable foods — and shop once a month at a warehouse or club store. Get your fresh foods and specialty items at the supermarket. Plan to do your main shopping once a week and run in a second time only if you need to pick up perishables. Try to limit your shopping at convenience stores. Though they're hard on your budget, convenience stores are oh-so-easy in emergency situations. Just be sure to buy only what the emergency requires — and the first time you find yourself there for toothpaste, add it to your backup list.

❀ **Shop at the right time.** Try to resist the urge to shop when you and the rest of the world want to most: just before dinner. You may be competing at the meat counter and standing in line forever — and you're likely to buy more when you're hungry. Morning and late evening make great grocery times in today's 24/7 environment, as does the day after your favorite store stocks its shelves (ask a friendly manager).

❀ **Shop in the right sections.** The hot service counter, salad bar, gourmet-sauce shelf, and prepared-foods section are great when you're in a hurry, not so good when you're on a budget.

Unloading the goodies

After grocery shopping, unloading efficiently can save time and stress. Keep a collapsible crate in the trunk of the car to help carry bags into the house. If you live in a high-rise building, a folding shopping cart can help you get your groceries upstairs with ease. Just remember to put the heavy items on the bottom, or they'll squish your vegetables and bread!

As you unload the groceries, be thinking about how and when each item can be used. Organizing as you unpack items can give you a head start on busy mornings and harried meal times. For instance, wash and ice the mini-carrots for the kids to snack on. Seal pretzels into resealable plastic bags to tuck into lunches. Toss out all those old and spoiled things you come across as you put away the new.

Cookbooks and Recipes

The recipes that tell you what to do for delicious success can be a source of vital sustenance and heritage — when they're not cluttering the kitchen

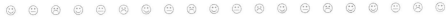

with information overload. Systematize your cookbooks and recipes into accessible references instead of acres of meaningless paper, and watch your culinary prowess soar.

Cleaning up your cookbook collection

Everybody needs at least one all-purpose cookbook, so whether you wonder what to do with the fresh Muscovy duck you just bought or are summoned to provide oatmeal cookies for the school bake sale, you have somewhere to turn. Beyond that, it's a question of how much you (really, actually) cook. Go through your cookbook collection and purge anything you haven't consulted or cooked from in a year, even if the book was a gift or a quaint collection from your local Junior League.

The library is well stocked with cookbooks for that special occasion when you need an appetizer from Ecuador. Resist the urge to buy new cookbooks you don't need. Store cookbooks in the kitchen, where they're used. You can contain them on a pantry shelf, install a shelf on the wall, or, if your collection is legitimately large, arrange them in a small freestanding bookshelf, grouped by type.

Reducing your recipe burden

Notice how recipe clippings just sort of fall out all over the place when you have to find a recipe? This calls for some action. Your step-by-step solution is as follows:

1   **Get two three-ring binders and a stack of plastic sheet protectors.**

2   **Sort your recipes into two piles: *to try* and *tried and true.***

    Toss out anything you tried and haven't loved, recipes you've lost interest in, recipes dated over a year back, or those so old the paper they're printed on has turned yellow.

3   **Write today's date on the recipes in the *to try* pile.**

4   **Slip recipes into sheet protectors, fitting in as many as you can see.**

    File the recipes, one pile per binder, according to sections marked with tabbed dividers — appetizers, meats, poultry, seafood, pasta, desserts, and so forth. Label the binder spines so you can distinguish the tried from the new. (See Chapter 14 for more information on setting up binders.)

☺ ☹ ☺ ☺ ☺ ☺ ☺ ☺ ☺ ☺ ☺ ☺ ☺ ☺ ☺ ☺ ☺ ☺ ☺ ☹ ☺

Voilà! Now you know just where to go to find your favorite no-cook pasta sauce or the hazelnut-crusted halibut recipe that looks so fabulous for your next dinner party.

Card files are a hard-work way to store recipes. You have to do amazing feats of origami to get the recipes clipped in a way that they fit on the card, or rewrite the whole thing from scratch. Try the binder approach and spare yourself the extra effort. To maintain your binders, throw away any recipe you try but don't like, and move those you do like into the *tried and true* binder. Date all new *to try* recipes as you file them, and toss them after they've sat around for a year. Chances are that the dishes don't really fit your lifestyle, and there are plenty of new ones coming.

If you're a serious cook and computer-savvy, you may want to consider filing your recipes on your computer, in special recipe software that also runs nutritional analyses and generates shopping lists, or in your word processing program. Recipe programs are set up to organize your recipes by section; if you use a word processor, create a different folder for each type of dish. Getting recipes entered takes extra time, but you save storage space and can print a fresh copy whenever you need one.

Coupons: Turn Clutter into Cash in Hand

When coupons are properly clipped, filed, and redeemed, they can be great money savers, especially for larger families. The trick is to be efficient enough that you don't spend more time than the money you save is worth.

Here's the plan:

1   Get a 4-x-6-inch file box (3 x 5 inches is too small for wider coupons).

2   Add tabbed dividers and label them by five categories: food, household items, paper goods, personal, and other (batteries, camera, office and school supplies, and so on).

3   Tackle your coupons as soon as they arrive — the Sunday paper is a good source — and clip items you commonly use, know you need, or genuinely want to try.

4   File your coupons by section, putting the newest ones in back and weeding out those that have expired.

5   Mark the coupons that you know you want to use on your shopping list, and then take the whole box along for the ride so you never leave one behind or miss an opportunity to double up with an in-store special.

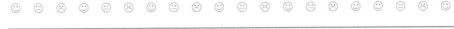

The cardinal rule for turning coupons into cash in hand is *don't clip anything you don't need.* When you shop, look for a place that redeems coupons at double their face value – usually large supermarkets, where you can do much of your drugstore shopping these days, too.

Store fast-food and take-out menus and coupons in a big (6-x-5-inch) magnetic pocket posted on the least-visible side of the refrigerator.

Sweeping the Kitchen Clean

Keeping the kitchen clean is a daily challenge, but with a few tricks up your sleeve you can create an almost self-cleaning kitchen. Here are some ideas for keeping daily kitchen cleanup organized and easy:

✸ **Wash up while you wait** for the water to boil, the chicken to roast, the sauce to reduce. Washing pots and pans as you use them leaves a smaller pile to clean up at the end.

✸ **Sweep after every meal,** or at least at the end of each day, so crumbs and fallen food don't get ground into the floor and make for a tough cleanup job later.

✸ **Keep your tools close by.** If you don't have a utility closet in the kitchen for the broom, dustpan, and mop, various organizers are available to hang them from a pantry wall. A first-floor laundry room is another place to put these implements.

✸ **Keep trash handy.** Most kitchens generate a great deal of garbage, so go ahead and get a nice big, plastic wastebasket that you won't have to empty every five minutes. Keep the wastebasket clean with a plastic garbage-bag liner, and watch for spills and mold in the bottom.

Chapter 4

The Ever-Popular Gathering Spot: The Family Room

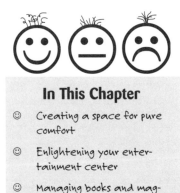

Though the family room is a great place to forget formality, that doesn't mean order can go out the window, too. Neatness counts extra in this room because it's usually the most lived-in. The den's image permeates the consciousness of your home's inhabitants. Wouldn't you like that picture to be one of peace?

Creating a P-L-A-C-E for Everyone

The model family room is comfort defined, a casual place for letting it all hang out. How can you let everyone do his or her own thing in the family room, yet still have some semblance of order? Teach all the room's occupants the power of the principles of P-L-A-C-E:

❀ **Purge:** Toss any malfunctioning, obsolete, or duplicate equipment; videos you no longer watch; music nobody listens to anymore; books you won't read again; and old magazines, including back issues you haven't read.

❀ **Like with like:** Arrange video- and audiotapes and discs by format and category, books by fiction/nonfiction and category, and photos by date in boxes or into albums or frames. Group remote controls together with a remote caddy.

☺ ☺ ☹ ☺ ☺ ☹ ☺ ☺ ☹ ☺ ☺ ☹ ☺ ☺ ☹ ☺ ☺ ☺ ☹ ☺

❈ **Access:** Arrange furniture for conversation, watching television, and listening to music. Place home-entertainment equipment in a media unit designed to accommodate units and make connections easy. In the bookcase, place heavier books on lower shelves and lighter ones higher up.

❈ **Contain:** Store and contain tapes and discs in drawers, shelves, or storage units, books in the bookcase, current magazines in a rack, and games, toys, photos, and collections in closed shelves and drawers or in the playroom or basement.

❈ **Evaluate:** Can you straggle into this room after a long, hard day and quickly access the recreation you crave? Is the room so comfortable and peaceful that you sometimes fall asleep in your chair? Do the members of your family get along, find what they need, and have fun when they're here?

Fun or Frustrating: The Media Center

A media unit is a must to provide easy access to a full complement of equipment — television, VCR or DVD, and stereo system. Designed to shelve the various components of your system and accommodate all the connecting cables, media units also have drawers to store manuals, pro- gram guides, cleaning kits, extra cables, tapes, and CDs. Built-in units offer the best stability, but you can also buy a free-standing system. If you must make do with a bookcase, drill holes in the back for cables and cords. Use extra shelf space and shelf-top organizers to store CDs and tapes.

The media center is the focal point of many family rooms — and face it, it tends to be a mess. If you accumulated a mass of unused entertainment equipment, clear the stuff out. The eight-track tape deck? History! The skipping CD player you keep thinking you'll take in for service? Either do it or give it away. Your little tabletop TV is shamed by the new big-screen model you just installed. Move the smaller version to the kitchen or call a charity for pickup.

TV, VCR/DVD, and stereo equipment

Does your remote control like to play hide-and-seek between the couch cushions? Take control with a caddy that has a place for your remote unit and current program guide. You can even attach it to your favorite easy chair. If you have several remotes for the television, video player, and stereo system, a universal unit can combine them all into one.

Fight media burnout with a scheme to make home entertainment easy again. Four easy steps can enlighten your entertainment collection and put hours of fun at your fingertips.

☺ ☹ ☹ ☺ ☹ ☹ ☺ ☹ ☹ ☺ ☹ ☹ ☺ ☹ ☹ ☺ ☹ ☹ ☺

1 **Gather the family and go through all your tapes and discs, purging everything that no one's watched or listened to for a year.**

Cries of extreme sentimental value can be accommodated, but remember that you can always rent videos as well as borrow movies and music from the library. As you go, sort items by like format — videotapes, video discs, audiotapes, and audio discs. If your cast-off CDs still have popular appeal, take them to a used CD store for cash. You can also donate CDs and commercial videos and audio-tapes to a library or school.

2 **Group like items by genre or category.**

Alphabetize titles within each category. Using the artist's or com-poser's name for audiotapes and the show name for videos is usu-ally the easiest method. Audio categories may include classical, jazz, rock/pop, rhythm and blues/soul, rap/hip hop, blues, country, musicals/soundtracks, world/folk, children's, and books on tape. For video, consider categorizing by movies, television shows, enter-tainment (concerts, magic shows), children's, sports, exercise, how-to, and home videos.

3 **Devise your optimal storage strategy by comparing your space to the number of pieces you need to store in each format and identifying where you can most easily reach them.**

Containing options for your audiovisual software include drawers (either in a media unit, a free-standing unit, or under coffee or end tables), shelves, spinning turntables, or free-standing towers.

4 **Identify your media.**

Make sure you have as much fun as your collection can offer with some basic media management. Create a computer list — a data-base, spreadsheet, or even just a word processing document — of everything in your collection by category. Keep an updated printout in a drawer of your media center as an easy-browsing menu. Label all video spines with program and length. Keep one videotape for each family member for recording favorite shows over and over. Label the tape with the individual's name and the show if it's always the same.

Just the highlights: Home video editing

Improve the production values of your home videos by editing as you shoot or later. When you first get a video camera, you'll probably go crazy taping your kids. But when they're all grown up, watching a video of a baby (even *your* baby) bouncing in a seat for 10 minutes straight probably won't be that fascinating.

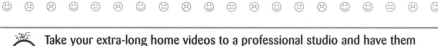

Take your extra-long home videos to a professional studio and have them edited down to highlights. This is also a great opportunity to have your old 8mm films and slides transferred to video so you can enjoy them more often. Just be sure to name, date, number, and log your originals before you let them out of your hands. Protect videos from getting erased by punching out the rerecord tabs.

The Computer Equation

In homes without an office, the family room may be the only place to put a computer. The downside of this strategy is that one family member may want to watch a movie or listen to mind-numbing heavy-metal music while another is trying to do homework or balance the checkbook on the computer. You may need to set rules — such as homework assignments come first. Having a spare TV in another room can help ease their enforcement. Use a chart like Table 4-1 to keep the family room on schedule and cut down on disputes.

Table 4-1 Family Room Schedule

Who?	What?	Where?	When?
Susan	Book report	Computer Workstation	Tues/Thurs 4–6 p.m.
Josh	Video games with friends	TV area	Friday 4:30–?

Managing Your Precious Moments: Photographs

The cherished memories in your photo collection can become a clutter problem fast. Shutterbugs can benefit from a few friendly photo tips. First, purge the lemons: There's no prize for hanging on to bad pictures, so give them the boot. After you've picked through and found all the ones that are blurry, too far away, or where the subject's eyes are shut, you can efficiently manage the ones that are worth keeping by doing the following:

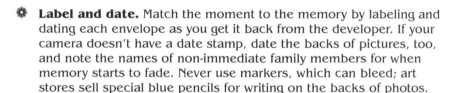

- **Label and date.** Match the moment to the memory by labeling and dating each envelope as you get it back from the developer. If your camera doesn't have a date stamp, date the backs of pictures, too, and note the names of non-immediate family members for when memory starts to fade. Never use markers, which can bleed; art stores sell special blue pencils for writing on the backs of photos.

- **Display.** What's the point of photos you never look at? Enjoy your pictures by putting them in frames or a photo album or scrapbook right away, or make a date with yourself to do it at least once a year (more if you're a frequent photographer). Some frames hold several pictures so that you can make your own collage. Have fun creating family history collages, and then hang them in the hall so everyone can remember where they came from.

- **Make scrapbooks.** Assembling a scrapbook is a great family project. Choose a snowy or rainy day, or if your kids are in college, steal a few hours over break. Check out scrapbook stores chock-full of things to jazz up your book, from funny quotes to fancy borders and stickers. If you prefer to seek professional help, there are specialists who teach design ideas and let you make multiple visits to their facility for advice and the camaraderie of other scrapbook creators.

- **Store safely.** Preserve your photos by keeping them in acid-free boxes or albums made with acid-free paper. Shoebox living can age photos fast.

Books and Bookshelves: The Library

You don't have to know the Dewey decimal system to bring order to your reading matter. Here's how to lighten up the library. Go through your books and purge all the dinosaurs, which include the following:

- Outdated or irrelevant reference books (such as the guide to colleges if all your kids have graduated).

- Novels you won't read again.

- Outgrown children's books.

- Old textbooks.

- Anything you don't expect to open in the next year (unless it's a classic). Information is now easy to access and quick to change, so don't clutter your bookcase with yesterday's news.

 Donate unwanted books to a library, school, or senior home, or sell your best titles to a used bookstore.

☺ ☺ ☹ ☺ ☺ ☹ ☺ ☺ ☹ ☺ ☺ ☹ ☺ ☺ ☹ ☺ ☺ ☺ ☹ ☺

Arrange your books on the shelves by category, grouping like with like. For fiction, you can categorize by novels, short stories, plays, and children's books. Good nonfiction categories include reference (dictionaries, encyclopedias, thesauruses), biography, history, religion, English, arts, science, math, health/medicine, crafts/hobbies, travel, photo albums, scrapbooks, and yearbooks. Ease access and be kind to your bookcase by keeping heavier books (think reference) on the bottom shelves and lighter ones (paperbacks) on top. Resist the urge to stack books two rows deep, because you may never see the ones in back. If you purged and still have more books than shelf space, it's time for a new bookcase. Look for one with adjustable shelves so you can change the height to suit hard covers or paperbacks.

Clutter or Current: Magazines

Magazines come out every week or month for a reason: You're supposed to read them now and move on. Keep only the current issues of magazines and purge the rest — yes, even if you haven't read them. If you later discover that you missed the only tell-all interview ever printed with your favorite movie star, you can find it at the library. (Schools sometimes use old magazines for various projects, if you'd rather donate than toss.)

Assess your subscription portfolio. Do you really need everything you receive? Is there a magazine you haven't gotten to for the last three issues? Are you reading some of them online? Do you subscribe to a weekly news magazine simply because you think you should only to have it lie around unopened week after week? Call to cancel any superfluous subscriptions.

The whole magazine: Rack 'em

Contain your current magazine issues in a rack. As each new issue arrives, rack it up and discard the previous one. No doubling up. You can use your magazine rack to store current catalogs, too. The same rule applies: Toss out the old as you rack up the new. If you receive catalogs you don't want, call and ask to be removed from the mailing list.

Articles: File 'em

For good magazine management, mark the table of contents of each issue as you get it and tear out any articles you want to read. (If you're sharing with others or like to browse the ads, you can pull the articles when the time comes to throw the magazine away instead.) Staple each article together and place it in a To Read file that you can take along on commutes, to the doctor's office, and so on. See Chapter 14 for more on how to filter information flow.

Games, Toys, and Collections

A family that plays together stays together, but how do you keep your fun neat? Most families accumulate quite a few games, toys, and collections in the course of having fun. You have to be fully equipped to play — you just need to give all your playthings a place.

Keeping games fun (and organized!)

If the family room is your prime game-playing area, buy a closed cabinet that can contain everything behind doors. A bookshelf is a less scenic alternative. Infrequent gamers or those just as likely to play in another room may put their gaming center in the playroom, basement, or hall closet, keeping just a couple of family favorites — cards, checkers — in a drawer in the den.

Keep electronic games by the TV on which they're played in clear storage boxes or special units designed to hold them.

The toy crate

Toys need to be mobile when you have toddlers so that you can keep the kids amused as you herd them around the house under your watchful eye. As long as your kids are little, keep a crate of toys in the family room so you don't have to chase up and down the stairs in search of a bear or truck. When the children are old enough to play in the playroom or their bedrooms without supervision, move the toys and eliminate the crate.

Part 2: Organizing Your Primary Living Spaces

☺ ☺ ☹ ☺ ☺ ☹ ☺ ☺ ☹ ☺ ☺ ☹ ☺ ☺ ☹ ☺ ☺ ☺ ☹ ☺

Chapter 5

Where the Creative Magic Happens: The Playroom

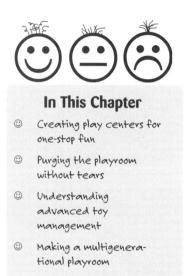

Play is important to people of all ages, but for children, amusement is a 24/7 job. The mess that can come from hard-core fun makes a separate room for play a great plan. Not only does a playroom keep toys, crafts, and games out from underfoot in the rest of the house, but a playroom also provides young minds with a special place to let their imaginations soar.

Using P-L-A-C-E in Your Playroom

Children learn as they play. Show your kids how to keep the playroom clean and organized, and you'll give them a powerful tool for productivity and clear thinking that can last a lifetime. P-L-A-C-E provides the framework for your cleaned-up playroom. Here's how you employ it:

❁ **Purge:** Throw away or donate outgrown, unused, and broken toys, including games and puzzles with missing pieces. Pitch old or duplicate-color crayons, dried-out markers, paints, and glue.

❁ **Like with like:** Put items into play centers — toddlers, dress-up, playing school, and so on. Place game pieces and puzzles into resealable bags and onto shelves. Arrange books by category.

❁ **Access:** Put all large equipment, such as indoor slides or train displays, at one end of the room, and potentially dangerous or messy art and craft supplies in a childproof cabinet near their use. Keep small toys such as marbles and doll accessories higher up, out of the reach of smaller children who can choke on them.

☺ ☺ ☹ ☺ ☺ ☹ ☺ ☺ ☹ ☺ ☺ ☹ ☺ ☺ ☹ ☺ ☺ ☺ ☺ ☹ ☺

❋ **Contain:** Place toys into containers by type and age group or individual. Add labels for quick identification and to help younger children learn to read. Put art and craft supplies into separate containers or rolling carts.

❋ **Evaluate:** Do children and adults feel free to play, create, and make believe in this room? Can children find and put away their own toys? Do games and puzzles always have all their pieces in place? Do you feel safe leaving your children here unsupervised? Is there a space for every sort of fun your family likes?

Positioning the Play Centers

The playroom can be conducive to creativity and to cleaning up afterward. Much of the action in this room takes place on the floor, so tackle that first and work your way up. A nice, soft carpet is great for ground-based games and play, but carpeting can also take a beating from art supplies and spills. A great solution is indoor/outdoor carpeting: Accidents can be vacuumed up or washed away with soap and water in a flash, and toys are easily pushed across the flat surface into piles for quick pickups. Genius!

Now for the fun part: Creating your worlds of play. You know how a grocery store stocks the pastas next to the sauces so you can pick up dinner all in one aisle? You can do the same in the playroom, setting up centers for various activities and age groups that make each spot a different adventure. Play centers are actually nothing more than an imaginative version of fingertip management and access, putting fun within easy reach.

One play center may include toddler toys, while another part of the room is set up to play school. The dress-up center can contain clothes and a mirror for showing them off; the building center could be stocked with builder sets; and the music center gathers together instruments, tapes and CDs, and players. If you have big equipment such as a slide or trampoline, establish an action center at one end of the room.

 Your play center arrangements may need to change with your children's interests and ages. Freshening up the playroom with periodic repositioning keeps everyone interested in its organization, and provides an excellent opportunity to purge the cast-offs as you go.

How to Be a Senior Toy Manager

If you've been there, you know: Toy management is serious business. Those who manage toys well ought to receive an honorable degree, acknowledging the advanced techniques required to keep order between fun-loving young souls and the adults who love to lavish them with gifts.

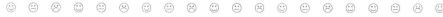
The good news is that when you master the three key toy-management principles, you can keep your playroom and its players on track without panicking every time the grandparents show up with presents.

The three steps to advanced toy management are:

1 Purge.

2 Contain.

3 Rotate.

Each of these steps is covered in more detail in the following sections.

Purge

In today's world, many kids are in total toy overload. To adults, toys can come to represent both love and money spent, and tossing toys may be even harder for mom than daughter. But as sentimental as each gift from loving parents, doting grandparents, and adoring aunts and uncles may be, kids outgrow toys quickly and can only play with so many current favorites at once. Keeping extra or obsolete toys encourages bad habits and wastes space — which itself is a critical part of the creativity equation. So take the plunge: Purge your playroom today.

Depending upon your children's ages and the toys involved, you may choose to approach the task with each child individually, or do the whole family in one fell swoop. Sort toys and games by type, directing the cast-offs to trash, donation, and garage-sale piles as you go.

You can approach purging your playroom gently. Never make children get rid of toys before they're ready, but do look for staged compromises that respect a child's feelings while also helping children form a healthy relationship with material things.

Contain

Enclosing toys in containers keeps them from becoming clutter and accustoms kids to looking for things in their place and putting their toys back in the appropriate container later.

Match the container to the type of toy and age of the users. Colored open crates can hold large toys for small toddlers. Use a different color for each type of toy — blocks, cars, dolls, animals.

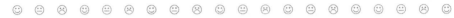

No cutting corners: Storing games

One nice thing about games is that they come in their own box, but boy do those boxes break fast, especially the corners. Mend breaks with masking tape applied to the inside of the box, which can keep the box looking nice and improve your chances of getting the game out and put away without pieces all over the floor.

Speaking of pieces, protect your peace of mind by zipping them into resealable bags. This makes cleanup far easier when the box takes a tumble. Use the slide type of closure for easy access to younger kids' games and a pressure closure for those you may want to keep little ones out of.

Some games have paper books that are necessary to play the game. If the game is a family favorite, extend the life of the book by covering the pages with clear contact paper.

Clear, pullout drawers suit smaller items and make seeing what's inside easy at play and cleanup time. Preschoolers love them. Closed wicker baskets or chests are an attractive way to house dolls and doll clothes. Containers with tight-fitting lids keep smaller children out of older children's toys, so that Judy can keep her beloved doll accessories in the playroom without worrying that little Phillip may stop by and swallow a tiny high-heeled shoe.

Arrange your containers in cabinets or on wall shelves, keeping crayons, board games, and craft supplies up high and toddler-friendly toys closer to the floor.

 Go for closed: Look for full backs and sides on all your playroom containers and shelving. Small toys and game and puzzle pieces have a way of slipping through cracks into irretrievable spots.

Rotate

Even after your purge, you'll probably have more toys than your children can play with at once. Absence makes the heart grow fonder, so prolong the appeal of toys and games by rotating your active stock.

 To establish a toy rotation, divide each toy type into a few different groups, so that the sum of one group from each type will leave your playroom well-stocked. Box up the remaining groups by set, label each "Toy rotation #___", and store in the basement or attic far from inquiring eyes. Make a quick toy inventory, like the one in Table 5-1 and keep it handy. That way you'll know what you have where.

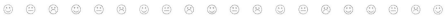
When your kids start to tire of the playroom repertoire, it's time for the big switcheroo. You can make a big deal of the switch, enlisting kids to pack up old toys before bringing on the new batch, or make the change yourself quietly one night. Surprise! Rotations also provide a good time to trim down the collection. Are all the toys you'll pack up still on the A list? Toss or donate the Cs through Zs — but remember that a little time away can reestablish the luster of many a B.

Table 5-1 Toy Inventory

Toy Rotation Box #	Key Items Contained	Box Location
Box #1	Annoying talking toucan, board games (Trouble, Sorry, Operation), shape sorter	Basement storage

Getting it together: Puzzles

You can never put all the pieces of a puzzle together if some have gone missing, so use a system to keep them in their place:

* As soon as you bring a puzzle home, mark the back of each piece with the puzzle's name or a number, for example, "Farmhouse" or "23." If you use a number code, write the number on the puzzle box. Now if a piece pops up somewhere else, you know just where to put the piece back.

* Put puzzle pieces into a resealable bag inside the box to prevent spills.

* Devote a card or snack table to the puzzle for as long as you work on it. Place the table in a corner to keep it from getting knocked over or interfering with other activities.

The Reading Center: Children's Books

Playrooms are often freewheeling places — not the best environment for a reading center, so I generally recommend keeping most children's books in bedrooms or the library or family room. However, the playroom is the right room for activity, art, and craft books, and you may put the rest of your collection here if you don't have space elsewhere or if the playroom is your prime reading spot. Depending upon how many books you have, use a small free-standing bookcase or larger wall unit to put them into place. If you keep reading books here, put older children's books higher up so younger siblings won't access and destroy them; devote the lower shelves to toddler favorites. Shelve books by like category: activity, reference, fiction or stories, fairy tales, religious books, and so on. See Chapter 4 for more on categorizing and shelving a library.

The Art of Organizing Arts 'n Crafts

Setting up an arts and crafts area for kids is like arranging an adult workshop or hobby area, while accounting for safety issues and a lot more messes.

First, create the art center. Remind yourself that if there's a nice carpet on the floor, you may want to recarpet with indoor/outdoor material, use a drop cloth, or relegate activities involving clay, paints, markers, or glue to the kitchen. Keep all messy supplies in a childproof cabinet closest to their use.

Getting a jump on reading while you play with labels

Even toy retrieval can become a reading experience when you label toy containers with their contents. Tommy may not know the word *cars* on sight, but show him that his toy hot rod goes in the drawer with those four letters on the front and watch his cognitive wheels start to turn.

Make the reading lesson easier by using both upper- and lowercase letters in your labels. Small letters, with their distinct shapes and heights, are easier to recognize than all caps. Use a label maker, which is relatively cheap (less than $50), for the job and the resulting labels look much better than masking tape or a curling computer label, and they're washable. With your help, your preschoolers may like punching out a label or two for themselves.

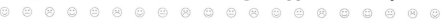
 If you don't have a mess-proof floor in the art center or want to double up your cooking with supervising an arts-and-craft session, set up your craft station in the kitchen, storing supplies in a high or locked cabinet and using the kitchen table for a worktable. You can knock off a stew or sauce while they stamp, paint, or glue, and everyone can have something to show at the end.

Buy washable markers, paints, and glue while kids are young enough to consider the world and the walls their canvas. For a worktable in the playroom, a kitchen cast-off fills the bill. Laminated tops are easiest to clean up, while wood may get wrecked and stained by paints and crayons, but maybe you don't care.

Next, stock your supplies. As always, art supplies can be accessible close to the worktable, with like items together and everything contained in dividers or other containers in drawers or on shelves. An old dresser may be put to use for craft supply storage. Playrooms have lots of craft stuff and art supplies, so here are some ways to consolidate and store all those supplies for those future creations:

* **Crayons:** Save new, intact boxes of crayons for school and collect the rest in a covered plastic box or metal tin at home. Metal won't get as marked up as plastic.

* **Pencils, pens, markers, scissors:** Use narrow plastic divider trays, preferably inside a drawer to prevent a spill.

* **Rubber stamps:** Store them in their original cases or spread on a piece of paper. Stamping the paper with the design can help you find the stamp you want.

* **Paints:** Stack watercolors in their own containers, organize others into plastic trays.

* **Glues:** Group together in a plastic tray.

* **Paper:** If you have several types (white, construction, drawing, and so on), use an office sort tray.

* **Beads:** Corral beads into containers specially designed to separate them by type.

 Attention kids and parents everywhere: Crayons aren't used up just because you wore them down to the paper. Buy a crayon sharpener to keep a slim tip on your crayons and enjoy their full lifespan. Got more crayons than you can use? Daycare centers are always happy for the donation.

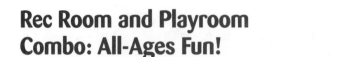

Rec Room and Playroom Combo: All-Ages Fun!

Everyone needs to play, and doubling up the playroom as a recreation and relaxation room for teenagers and adults can be a boon to family togetherness — if you have the space to let everyone do their thing. Keep centers in mind so that you can cohabitate playfully and peacefully. Add an adult sitting area with a couch, some comfy chairs, and perhaps a media center and/or library. Big games such as pool or Ping-Pong can go into their own game center away from the sitting area so the action doesn't detract from anyone's relaxation factor. Point the couch and chairs toward the kids' play areas, and you can keep a watchful eye while you enjoy your book or show.

Cleaning up your act

The playroom may be the space with the shortest organizational attention span in the house. Whatever the project or game, every session here needs to routinely end with cleanup time. From the moment your children can walk, show them not to walk out of the room until everything is put away. The payoff? Fun and easy play tomorrow, without a mess to wade through on the way.

Kid-friendly ways to clean up your act include the following:

❀ Clean up with them when the kids are young.

❀ Invite older children to think up better ways to straighten up and systematize the playroom. Throw down the gauntlet anew every year.

❀ Turn on special cleanup music and challenge everyone to be done by the time the song is over.

❀ Set a good example yourself in other areas of the house. Getting organized in the playroom can make fun come naturally for all.

Chapter 6

Tending to Toiletries: The Bathroom

In This Chapter

- Improving your grooming with P-L-A-C-E
- Defusing bathroom danger zones
- Getting a medicine cabinet Rx

Getting organized in the bathroom can make your mornings go faster and the nightly beeline for bed easier. Perfect your look by arranging all your toiletries within fingertip reach, and polish up your image with well-ordered facilities you can present to guests and visiting repair people without shame. With beautiful bathrooms, organization gets personal.

Where Order Meets Indulgence

Tackle the bathrooms one at a time. You may start with the master bath for inspiration; move on to the family bathroom, where you have your work cut out for you; and finish up with a finesse to the guest baths. In each room, select one section at a time — the countertop, cabinets, drawers, shower and bath, or linen closet and use the five-step P-L-A-C-E system to whip everything into shape and beautify your bathroom space.

- **Purge:** Toss odds and ends of soap and old, worn, or excess washcloths, towels, sheets, sponges, scrubbers, and loofahs. Eye shadow, lipstick, and blush more than two years old; foundation and powder more than one year old; and eyeliner or mascara more than six months old are neither hygienic nor high quality anymore. So throw them away, along with any personal-care products that you haven't used in the last year. Check dates on medications and dispose of expired ones. Are you using all those travel products collected on your trips? If not, out they go. Old or extra magazines can move to the family room or the trash.
- **Like with like:** Organize personal-care items and supplies by type in your cabinet drawers, underneath the cabinet, or on linen-closet shelves. Shower and bath items can be kept on standing or hanging racks sorted by type or by person.

❀ **Access:** Place items close to where they're used but out of bathroom users' way, considering safety issues if children are in the house. Countertop items can move to the medicine cabinet, drawers, and under-sink cupboards. Medications need a cool, dry shelf out of the reach of small kids.

❀ **Contain:** Use baskets, drawers, and/or drawer dividers to contain items by like type: cosmetics, personal-care products, medicines, hair accessories, nail supplies. Put anything that can spill in a leak-proof container. Label containers so putting things back from where they came from is easy.

❀ **Evaluate:** Can you find everything you need to get ready on the sleepiest morning and get to bed on a dog-tired night? Can you shave, style your hair, and apply makeup without taking a step? Is keeping the guest bathroom neat enough for strangers easy?

The Organizational Conundrum: Sink and Vanity

Though different people may frequent the master and family bathrooms, you can apply the same logic to both. As always, finish one room before moving on to the next.

If you have a nice, big counter alongside your sink, count yourself lucky and then count up how much stuff is cluttering the space. Things left on the countertop look messy, attract dust, and get in the way of your grooming routines. Here's what can stay out on your sink or countertop:

❀ Hand soap

❀ Drinking glasses

❀ Box of tissues

❀ Clock (Put it on the wall if you can!)

For the rest of your countertop display, put everything away closest to where you usually access it. Elegant perfume bottles can grace a bureau in the bedroom. Shaving supplies go into a cabinet or drawer, along with cosmetics, hair products, and bath things. Slip the blow dryer down below, under the sink.

If your bathroom scores low on drawers and you have a clear corner on the counter, get a set of small countertop drawers to keep your cosmetics and hair accessories neat and invisible. Figure 6-1 shows this sleight-of-hand. (Consider safety if children visit this bathroom.)

☺ ☺ ☹ ☺ ☺ ☹ ☺ ☺ ☹ ☺ ☺ ☹ ☺ ☺ ☹ ☺ ☺ ☺ ☹ ☺

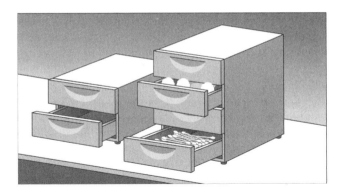

Figure 6-1: Countertop drawers expand your options for storage.

Photo courtesy of Get Organized!

Locate your wastebasket near the sink so tossing out tissues, cotton balls, and razor blades is easy. Plastic is best for bathroom trash bins; a bag lining keeps the wastebasket clean and protects it from corrosive agents such as nail-polish remover.

Medicine cabinet: A misnomer

Whoever named the medicine cabinet must have had excellent health because the medicine cabinet is a terrible place to keep any kind of medication for three reasons:

❀ **Safety:** This cabinet is all too accessible to children. Keep small stomachs safe from the dangers of all medications, from aspirin to iodine, by storing them on high or locked shelves.

❀ **Spoilage:** Heat and humidity from the shower and bath can quickly dissipate the potency of drugs and dietary supplements. Head for drier, cooler ground.

❀ **Accessibility:** Many medications are meant to be taken with food. Unless you eat breakfast in the bathroom, that would put their closest use in the kitchen.

Now that you have the shelves cleared out, here's how to fill them up. Most medicine cabinets have three removable shelves that slide into slots of varying heights. If you have such adjustable architecture, match altitude to access by making the top shelf the highest to fit tall items. That leaves smaller things for the lower shelves, where you can easily spot them, and the shortest for the middle shelf. Here is an example:

❀ **Top shelf:** Hair spray, gel, mousse, shaving cream, aftershave, cologne, antiperspirant, mouthwash

☺ ☺ ☻ ☺ ☺ ☻ ☺ ☺ ☻ ☺ ☺ ☻ ☺ ☺ ☻ ☺ ☺ ☺ ☺ ☻ ☺

❋ **Middle/shortest:** Toothpaste and toothbrushes, dental floss, razor and refill blades

❋ **Bottom/medium height:** Facial cleansers and lotions, makeup remover and pads, contact lens supplies, eye drops, nasal spray

---

 Do you really want a day's worth of dust on something you put in your mouth? If not, skip the countertop display and hang your toothbrushes from slots in a medicine cabinet shelf instead. Get a different color brush for each bathroom user, and then write down the color code, noting the date the brush was put in service to remind you to replace it six months later. Make your own, or copy and tape Table 6-1 inside your medicine cabinet.

Table 6-1 Keeping Track of Toothbrushes

Brand	Color	Date in Service
_____	_____	_____
_____	_____	_____
_____	_____	_____
_____	_____	_____
_____	_____	_____
_____	_____	_____
_____	_____	_____

Dividing it up: Drawers

Divide your bathroom drawers for fingertip management of the snarl of items commonly found there. Dividers can range from 2-x-2-inch plastic trays up to full-drawer sectioned trays. Special cosmetics dividers are designed to hold lipsticks, eye shadows, and so forth; others are sized to hold jewelry. Measure your drawers, count your categories, and shop.

Got just one bathroom drawer? Unless you're a guy, this is probably the place for cosmetics and basic hair tools. Slip in hair accessories if they fit. A rolling cart of drawers is a great addition when you're short on built-ins. It works and it moves. See Table 6-2 for using bathroom drawer space effectively.

Storing: Under-the-sink cabinets

The space under the sink is a primary storage area for most bathrooms but because shelves are rare in these cabinets, pandemonium is all too common. Solve this problem with space-expanding options:

Table 6-2 Divine Bathroom Drawers

Drawer	Items
Cosmetic center	Foundation, blush, lipstick, eyeliner and shadow, mascara, sponges, brushes, tools
Hair care center	Comb, brush, headbands, barrettes, clips, hairpins, bobby pins, ponytail holders
Jewelry center	Earrings, necklaces, bracelets, watches, pins, jewelry cleaner, polishing cloth

- ✸ **Wire-coated shelves** are a quick, no-installation way to add a level to your cabinet. Buy the stackable or multi-tiered sort if you have lots of vertical space.

- ✸ **Pullout shelves** slide out of the cabinet to save you from having to reach inside.

- ✸ **Add a shelf** by buying a piece of wood to size and nailing it in. You may want to make your shelf half the cabinet's depth to leave room for tall things in front.

- ✸ **Hang a caddy** inside the cabinet door for hair dryers and curling irons. Check out Figure 6-2, and don't forget to account for clearance space.

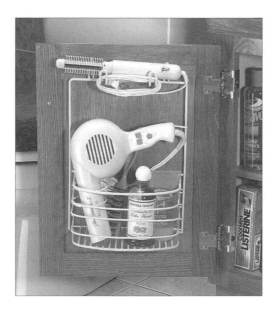

Figure 6-2: Cabinet door caddy for hair dryer, curling iron, detangler, and brushes.

Photo courtesy of Get Organized!

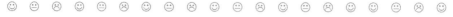
Next, group your items by like type to create under-sink centers and contain them in clear containers or baskets. Table 6-3 shows you how.

Table 6-3 Under-Sink Centers

Centers	Items
Hair-care center	Dryer, curling iron, straightener, crimper
Nail-care center	Manicure set, nail polish, polish remover, pads
Feminine-hygiene center	Tampons, pads, freshness products
Sun-protection center	Sunscreen, self-tanner, after-sun moisturizer (move to the linen closet for off-season storage)
Cleaning-supply center (if no small children are in the house)	Scouring powder, spray cleanser, glass cleaner, disinfectant, toilet-bowl cleaner
Plumbing center	Plunger, drain unclogger

If your bathroom serves a large family, get each person a different colored basket to stow personal things in the under-sink cabinet.

Medications made simple and safe

Whether you pop a multivitamin once a day or take a complicated regime of pills by the hour, a well-managed medication system can make a big difference to your health:

* **Store safe and smart.** Keep all medications out of the reach of children, away from the heat and humidity of the bath, and closest to where you take them. This may mean that your daily dose goes into a kitchen cabinet for swallowing after meals, while allergy medicines are stored on the top shelf of the linen closet.

* **Group medications by like type.** Pain relievers, stomach remedies, sleep aids, and supplements may be located in different places according to the rule of access.

* **Stay up-to-date.** Check the expiration dates on both prescription and over-the-counter medications and pitch them when their time has come (usually a year).

* **Keep it straight.** If you take several medications each day, pill boxes with slots for each dose can make life much easier and prevent potentially dangerous mishaps.

* **Be prepared for emergencies.** Keep a bottle of Syrup of Ipecac in your first-aid kit to induce vomiting in the event of poisoning or dangerous drug reactions. Post the number of your local emergency room on the fridge or close to the phone.

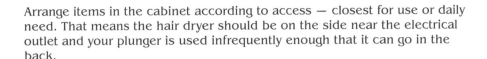

Arrange items in the cabinet according to access — closest for use or daily need. That means the hair dryer should be on the side near the electrical outlet and your plunger is used infrequently enough that it can go in the back.

Anything that overflows from your bathroom cabinet space can go in the linen closet, if you have one. Coming up short? Try the following:

✽ Try the various shelving or cabinet units that go above the toilet or stand freely on the floor. Some even have wheels for maximum mobility.

✽ Open shelves look cluttered, so contain items when you can — including a toilet paper holder that conceals extra rolls while keeping them close at hand, and a container to hold the toilet brush.

✽ If you like to have reading material within reach, get a basket or magazine rack to hold up to a half-dozen magazines.

Shower and Bath

If you have the same sort of array of personal-care products in your bath or shower and piles of towels all around that I see in my clients' homes, you're well aware of the problem that cleanliness presents: more supplies than space.

Where to hang the towels

For each person, install a towel bar that can hold a washcloth, hand towel, and bath towel. Towel bars are easy to add to a bathroom and can keep towels off the floor and other people from snatching yours. One person can use the shower-door bar if you don't have a bath mat hanging there; the back of the door provides another bar-hanging spot. For big families in small bathrooms, double up the hand and bath towel to squeeze two people onto one bar if you have to. Another space-saving option for a bathroom with four or more users is the towel bar that hangs on the door hinge.

Personal-care products and bath toys

Every shower and bath needs storage systems to hold shampoo, conditioner, skin cleansers, brushes, scrubbers, loofahs, razors, and shaving cream. These can take the form of corner shelves, a rack that hangs from the showerhead, or a tension-rod pole that extends from the top of a bathtub to the ceiling. Depending upon the size of your family, you can assign shelves by like products or by person.

First-aid center: Safety first

A complete first-aid center can be a quick, sometimes critical help for illnesses and injuries, but many of its contents can be poisonous or dangerous to small children. Prevent your own first-aid emergency by keeping your kit on a high linen-closet shelf.

The components of a well-stocked first-aid center may include: adhesive bandages, gauze pads and adhesive tape, elastic bandages, arm sling, ice bag, heating pad, antibiotic ointment, muscle-sprain cream, rubbing alcohol, hydrogen peroxide, calamine lotion, sunburn products, thermometer, scissors, tweezers, aspirin (or ibuprofen/acetaminophen for children), antihistamines, loperamide, bismuth, Syrup of Ipecac, and prescription insect-bite or food-allergy kits.

Rather bathe than shower? You may want all your supplies on hand without standing up to reach the soap, so get a tray that fits across the width of the tub to hold bath essentials. Some come with a book holder, so you can relax and read without worrying about your best-seller getting wet.

Next take on the rubber duckies: Put kids' bath toys in a mesh bag and hang it from the faucet. If the bath toys don't fit, you have too many . . . *unless* you have a baby, whose toys are often super-size. Keep those in a dishpan that goes in the under-sink cabinet or floor of the linen closet between baths.

Hand washables solution: No wet stuff draped on the towels

Doing small hand-wash jobs in the bathroom may be more convenient than trudging down to the laundry room, but lingerie draped all over is not an attractive sight. Get a closed, nontransparent hamper to hold hand-wash items until washing day, and then dry them on a wire grid rack that hangs over the showerhead, a horizontal rack that sits inside or across the bathtub (this rack is great for sweaters too), or an old-fashioned folding wooden drying rack.

The Half or Guest Bath

Bath math dictates that you can have only half the stuff in a guest bath as in a main bathroom:

Chapter 6: Tending to Toiletries: The Bathroom

😊 😐 🙁 😊 😐 🙁 😊 😐 🙁 😊 😐 🙁 😊 😐 🙁 😊 😊 😐 🙁 😊

✱ **Sink and counter:** Maximize the aesthetics of the guest bath by keeping only what visitors may need out on the countertop. Sink and counter items may include a decorative pump-style bottle of liquid soap (so that guests don't have to share germs), a box of tissues, a bottle of hand lotion, and some small paper cups.

✱ **Towel bar:** Hang at least two hand towels in the guest bath.

✱ **Under-the-sink cabinet:** This is the spot for hiding away necessities and supplies, such as an extra package of toilet paper, box of tissues, bottle of hand soap, and feminine-hygiene supplies. Some cleaning supplies to have here are sponges, scouring powder, spray cleanser, glass cleaner, toilet-bowl cleaner, and a plunger.

✱ **Reading material:** Keep magazines neat with a small stand and don't overfill.

Now you're all cleaned up in your cleanup centers. Doesn't your bathroom feel beautifully pristine?

☺ ☻ ☹ ☺ ☻ ☹ ☺ ☻ ☹ ☺ ☻ ☹ ☺ ☻ ☹ ☺ ☺ ☻ ☹ ☺

Chapter 7

I'll Take a Few Extra Zzzz's: Bedrooms

In This Chapter

☺ Making your bedroom a great escape

☺ Keeping kids' rooms clutter-free

☺ Getting the most from your guest room

Quick — in what room of the house do you spend the most time? Even if you're a true couch potato commonly found glued to the tube in the TV room, a committed gourmet cook who can't stay out of the kitchen, or a perennial socialite spotted every night holding court in the living room, just about everyone but an insomniac spends most of his time at home in the bedroom catching up on sleep. Experts say we're *supposed* to sleep a third of our lives away, and everything you do in the room dedicated to relaxation can be extra sweet when you set it up as a personal and peaceful retreat.

Practicing P-L-A-C-E in the Bedroom

To get started in bringing balance to your bedrooms, select where you want to begin: yours, the kids', or the guest bedroom. If you want, skim the headings of the following sections to target a problem area, or simply work your way through the chapter to put everything in its place. In fact, P-L-A-C-E sums up the steps that see you, start to finish, through the race.

❀ **Purge:** Donate or toss clothes, broken, unused, or outgrown toys, accessories, jewelry, and perfume you haven't worn or used in more than a year. Pitch kids' old artwork and papers. (Yes, you can save some! Read on.)

❀ **Like with like:** Organize clothes by type, style, and color. Group shoes, purses, scarves, and ties by color.

❀ **Access:** Stock your bedside table with everything you need to make it through the night. Move the clothes you wear most frequently to top drawers and the closest parts of the closet, using tiers to double the number of items within reach. Find a shoe organizer that works with your space. Move off-season clothes to another closet or storage area, desk and papers to the office, extra books and tapes to the family room, extra toys and games to the playroom, and kids' papers that you want to keep in a memory box in the storage area. For the full story on closets, check out Chapter 11.

❋ **Contain:** Put jewelry into jewelry boxes, men's accessories into valet trays, underwear and socks into drawer dividers, and shoes and accessories into organizers. Arrange books in bookcases and organize toys into crates, drawers, baskets, or containers with lids.

❋ **Evaluate:** Do you start to relax as soon as you walk through the bedroom door? Can you crawl into bed, enjoy your favorite relaxing pursuit, and sleep through the night without getting up? Do you wake up refreshed? Can you pull together great outfits and accessories — even in the dark? Do children sleep and play in their rooms happily and safely?

Master Bedroom

It's not just for sleeping anymore. Once considered a crash pad in which the bed was the primary focus, many adult bedrooms now double as a private place to relax, far from the blaring TV or boisterous kids. Organizing this room can send you to sleep more satisfied and calm, make opening your eyes each morning a pleasure, and provide sanctuary from the stress and strain of life.

Arranging your bedroom

With big items like beds and dressers to place and plenty of closets, doors, and windows to confuse the issue, arranging furniture for optimal bedroom function can be an architectural challenge. That's why you need a blueprint. Use these principles to bring order to your bedroom with the following steps:

1 **Sketch your bedroom to scale according to the instructions in Chapter 2.**

2 **Survey the possibilities of what to put in your bedroom.**

Make sure you have the must-haves, and consider whether any additional options may suit your personal needs or help to streamline the room.

Must have: Bed, one or two night tables, one or two lamps, one or two dressers, a mirror, and a closet or armoire.

Optional: Built-in under-bed drawers, a headboard with a bookcase or cabinets, bookcase, media cabinet, reading chairs, and closet storage units and/or shelving.

☺ ☺ ☹ ☺ ☺ ☹ ☺ ☺ ☹ ☺ ☺ ☹ ☺ ☺ ☹ ☺ ☺ ☺ ☹ ☺

3 **Measure the big stuff — the bed, dressers, bookcase, media cabinet, armoire, and mirror — and make the cutouts described in Chapter 2.**

4 **Play with your layout.**

Look for where you can optimize your space according to the principles of fingertip management and access. If you're part of a couple, think of drawing an invisible line down the middle of the bed, and then arrange each partner's night table and dresser on his or her side.

Are two of you sharing a single bedside table, alarm clock, and reading lamp? Keep the peace with a pair of each situated on your respective sides. You'll both rest easier! (The same goes for your dresser, too.)

5 **Roll up your sleeves and put the furniture into place.**

Finishing touches may include a full-length mirror on the back of the door, and a small wooden or wicker chest at the foot of the bed to contain extra blankets that don't fit in the linen or bedroom closet.

Making the great escape

Because bedrooms aren't just for sleeping anymore, why not turn yours into a personal escape that satisfies your every need? Check the following list for suggestions:

❀ Add a great reading chair with an overhead lamp and a small bookcase or end table to make the bedroom an anytime retreat. Insomniacs should skip reading in bed, so a nice recliner can provide a solution for the sleepless.

❀ Do you like to watch your favorite show all snuggled up? Does music play a part in your love life, relaxation routine, or morning wake-up? Add a small media unit to your bedroom and organize the equipment, tapes, and discs according to the principles in Chapter 4. Closed cabinets are better than open shelves for storing media in the bedroom, where you want the picture to be purely peaceful. Keep the remote controls in your bedside table drawer so you don't have to drag yourself out of bed to skip a track or flick off the power.

❀ Arrange your boudoir for amour by clearing out all the workaday distractions and setting the mood with some strategically placed scented candles. Have your favorite soft-and-sultry CD ready to go and spray your pillows lightly with your favorite scent, unless somebody's allergic!

Stocking the amenities: Bedside table and dresser

Never does fingertip management seem as important as after you've crawled into bed, when a trip across the room for a pen takes on all the appeal of a trek to Siberia. For easy access, stock your bedside table with everything you need to get through the night so that you can sleep tight.

Start with a table that has drawers and/or shelves underneath to contain nightly necessities. On the tabletop go a reading lamp and alarm clock, and perhaps a radio or tape/CD player if you don't have a stereo in the room, a white-noise machine if it helps you sleep, and a coaster for a mug of tea or glass of water. The top drawer or shelf can hold a book or magazine, remote controls, eyeglasses, eye pillow or shade, pen and paper, a flashlight, and a travel alarm clock in case the power goes out.

Additional shelves or drawers can hold books and audiovisual disks or tapes. Select only your bedroom favorites and keep the rest with your main media center and library.

 Middle-of-the-night ideas can be brilliant, but they can also keep you up all night if you don't put them to rest. Keep a pen, small pad of paper, and flashlight in your night table so you can jot down anything from what your spouse should bring home from the store tomorrow to a quantum physics equation and get back to counting sheep. Some pens have built-in flashlights to assist your nighttime scribbling.

Main event: The dresser

Whether you call it a dresser, bureau, or chest of drawers, besides the bed, the dresser is the most important piece of furniture in the bedroom. How neat or messy it is governs how quickly, efficiently, and painlessly you can put yourself together on a groggy morning. The challenges with the dresser are twofold: Organizing everything you put in it and keeping the top clutter free. Like all surfaces, dresser tops too easily become storage areas. Don't let it happen. Here's what can stay out:

❀ Jewelry box(es)

❀ Perfume tray

❀ Valet tray

❀ One or two framed photos if you must, but why not hang them on the wall instead?

Find homes for everything else in drawers.

Boxing it up: Jewelry

Dazzling diamonds or simple silver chains, your jewelry needs to be in its place so you can find the right pieces to polish off your look. Are you storing some of your jewelry in its original boxes? Much as you may like the feel of the Ultrasuede or remembering that the bracelet came from Bloomingdale's, individual boxes waste space and hide their contents from your hunting eye. Take out what's inside and toss the containers. *Exception:* You can keep jewelry in its original box for storage in a fireproof or safe-deposit box.

☺ ☺ ☹ ☺ ☺ ☹ ☺ ☺ ☹ ☺ ☺ ☹ ☺ ☺ ☹ ☺ ☺ ☺ ☹ ☹ ☺

Now, box on a bigger scale. Unless you buy one of those big, expensive jewelry chests, chances are you won't find one box that holds your entire jewelry collection, but two should do (three if you have a lot). Match the shape and size of each box to what you keep inside. For necklaces, look for one with a horizontal bar and sprockets for hanging. You'll also find circular sprockets for long chains and necklaces, either as a separate container or on the sides of a jewelry box with drawers. If you don't have enough depth to hold bulky bracelets or earrings, buy a separate container for them.

If you're lucky enough to have the drawer space, you can get your jewelry off the dresser top by buying sectioned units that stack, sorting into the slots by like type and style, and keeping them inside drawers.

Don't let dust cloud the brilliance of your jewelry or perhaps increase the risk of infection in pierced ears. Skip the open-air ring displays and earring trees and contain everything inside a box or drawer.

Protect your most valuable jewelry from theft, fire, and disappearing down some mysterious crack by keeping it in a safe-deposit box at the bank. Before you go, get your jewels appraised and add a rider to your home insurance policy to cover them against loss or theft. Keep a list of what's in the safe-deposit box tucked into your jewelry box. Check out Table 7-1 for help in creating your own jewelry inventory. It's great for insurance purposes and peace of mind.

Table 7-1 Jewelry Inventory

Item	Description	Value	Location
Tennis bracelet	Princess cut diamonds set in gold	$2,500	Safe-deposit box

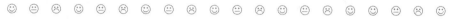

Men's accessories: Tray chic

Men may wear fewer adornments on average than women, but that doesn't mean they don't need a place to put them. A valet tray, which can range from a simple flat tray to a more elaborate affair with a drawer can help in holding on to little things such as:

❀ Tie bars

❀ Cuff links

❀ Watches

❀ Wallets

❀ Change

❀ Pins

❀ Pocket pens or pencils

❀ Pocket appointment books or electronic organizers

For infrequently worn items, choose a tray with a drawer to keep them out of the dust.

Now that you have the top all figured out and you're feeling a sense of accomplishment, take on the nitty-gritty of dresser usage and organization. What you put into the dresser is just as important as where you put it. Here is where organizing your wardrobe really begins! This piece of furniture is the place to keep the following items:

❀ Exercise clothes

❀ Nylons and tights

❀ Shorts

❀ Socks

❀ Sweaters (hanging them stretches the shoulders)

❀ Swimwear

❀ Thermal underwear

❀ T-shirts and tank tops

❀ Underwear and lingerie

Drawer management

Separate dressers are best if you share the bedroom. If you must share the bureau, too, designate separate drawers for each person.

Allocate items among drawers by putting like things together and the least frequently accessed items in the bottom drawers. No, thermal underwear

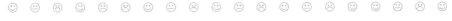

doesn't go with your slips just because you wear them both next to your skin. How often do you pull on long johns, and when do you ever add a slip on top? Put the thermals down below. Likewise, exercise hounds may want to keep their workout togs in a top drawer, but couch potatoes shouldn't bury them in the bottom as an excuse not to move!

Close to you: Innerwear

Your delicate items like to be handled with a soft touch, so start by dedicating one drawer to underwear and another to just nylons and slips. Next, add dividers so you can find the undergarment you need with ease. The soft, padded lingerie boxes pictured in Figure 7-1 are a nice alternative to the thin, hard plastic kind. Another option is a drawer divider.

 If you like to wear pantyhose under pants, keep a few pairs with inconspicuously placed runs. Use a permanent marker to write an *X* on the waistband and store them separately from your good ones.

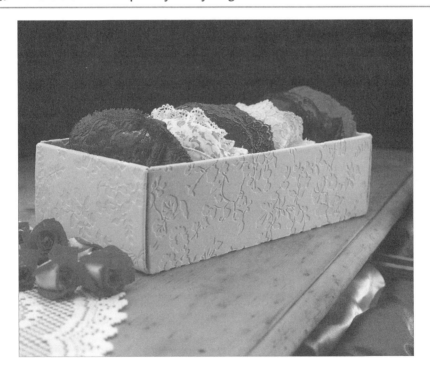

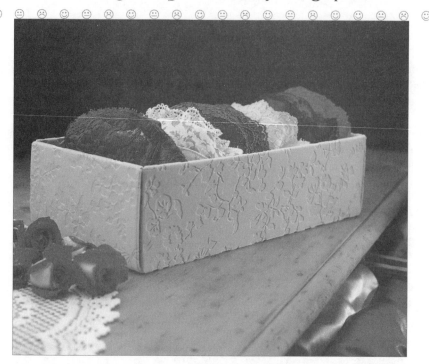

Figure 7-1: Keep lingerie straight and snag-free with soft, padded boxes.

Photo courtesy of Stacks and Stacks

Matched pairs and lost mates: Socks

Often a mess and unmatched to boot, socks need some help staying straight in the drawer. Here are my favorite sock-it-to-'em strategies:

❀ **Fold and stack.** Fold each pair in half together and put them on top of each other in neat stacks.

❀ **Wrap and toss.** For a more free-form approach, wrap one sock around the other into a little ball and toss it in the drawer. Nifty as this trick is, it can also stretch out the outer sock.

❀ **Divide.** Install a drawer divider, either a system of snap-together flexible polymer strips that gives each pair its own slot, or parallel dividers that run from the front to the back of the drawer.

❀ **Color code.** Use the front-to-back dividers so that you have a single lane of socks, and then arrange it by contrasting color — black at one end, brown at the other, and white in the middle. Navy, gray, and green can go by the whites, or start a separate row if you have enough. With precise color placement, you can match socks to pants in the dark, or at least through a colorblind morning haze. Still, do a final check before you walk out the door.

See Figure 7-2 for a view of these sock-taming techniques.

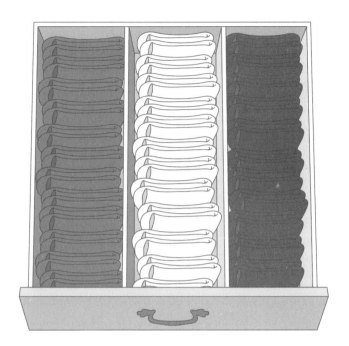

Figure 7-2: Drawer dividers keep socks in line.

Children's Bedrooms

Kids' bedrooms are multipurpose spaces, sort of a small person's living room, family room, and office all wrapped up in one. Children may play, listen to music or watch TV, do homework, or entertain friends for hours on end in their rooms, so having a setup that serves all these purposes without ending up a mess is important. Hey, it doesn't hurt to dream!

Kid-friendly furniture

Children grow quickly, and many parents fail to plan far enough ahead when furnishing their bedrooms. Spare yourself replacing big pieces as often as you do overalls by keeping the future in mind. As toddlers move out of cribs and into a regular bed, bypass the cutesy options and invest in a nice bedroom set.

Wide open space is at the top of kids' priority lists, so line up beds and furniture along the walls to leave plenty of room to play. Some children

☺ ☺ ☹ ☺ ☺ ☹ ☺ ☺ ☹ ☺ ☺ ☹ ☺ ☺ ☹ ☺ ☺ ☺ ☹ ☺

outgrow this need and will want to rearrange the furniture for a different look later.

For dressers and night tables, apply the same general principles you used in the master bedroom. If two siblings share a room, having separate tables and dressers situated near their owner's bed is best.

Books and toys

I think every child's bedroom should include a bookcase. Not only does it help keep everything in its place, but books in the bedroom can make reading a daily habit from the get-go. Bookcase needs may expand as a child grows and goes from a small collection of picture books to popular series, novels, reference books, and textbooks.

If there are so many toys in your child's bedroom that you have a hard time spotting the human being among them, it's time for a cleanup. Start with a purge of outgrown or redundant toys, which you may conduct in partnership with your child depending on age. Next, relocate what you can, using the playroom, if you have one, for primary toy storage and putting games with your family game center in the basement, hall closet, or family room. Then, contain what's left. See Chapter 5 for ideas on toy storage.

If you're wrestling with 20 to 30 stuffed animals when dusting or making the bed, tame the wild menagerie with a mesh hammock that drapes between two wall corners, or a plastic clip chain that hangs straight down from the ceiling. As you can see in Figure 7-3, the net needs a clear corner with no windows or closets in the way.

☺ ☺ ☹ ☺ ☺ ☹ ☺ ☺ ☹ ☺ ☺ ☹ ☺ ☺ ☹ ☺ ☺ ☺ ☹ ☺

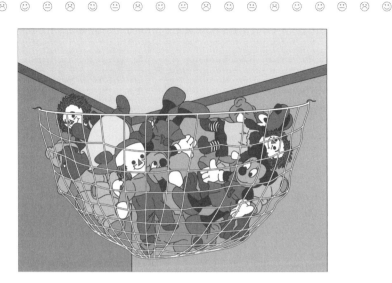

Figure 7-3: One way to tame your stuffed animal zoo.

From gold stars to watercolors: Papers

Kids become paper-making machines much earlier than you may think, and you need to exercise the same vigilance with their artwork, compositions, and stories that you do with your own paper flood.

One good place for papers in the bedroom is a bulletin board for junior-high students on up. Juggling school calendars and snapshots of friends, kids can benefit from a bulletin board that serves as a personal information center and a place to put visual mementos of the moment. Don't use metal thumbtacks that can land tack-side up. The colored plastic ones always fall sideways and are easier to find on the floor. Get your children thinking clear early on by limiting bulletin board contents to what fits without overlapping. If you want to add something new, something old must come down!

Guest Bedroom

Having a guest bedroom is a hospitable gesture, but this room can be a waste of space if you don't put it to double-duty. Set up right, the guest bedroom can make friends and family comfortable when they visit and serve other functions all the other days of the year. The guest bedroom closet may be storing your off-season clothes, but leave enough space for visitors to hang their things, too, and have some spare hangers at the ready. Providing a place to put non-hanging items such as underwear, paja-

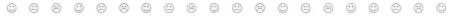
mas, and swimsuits is also thoughtful. A small chest of drawers does the trick; leave the top two drawers empty and dedicate the rest to the room's other use. Additional uses for your guest bedroom may include

❁ Entertainment or reading room

❁ Playroom

❁ Exercise room

❁ Sewing room

❁ Hobby room

❁ Home office

If you're using the room in other ways, a sofa bed saves space and provides a nice place to sit. Make sure there's room to open up the bed without moving furniture. No heavy coffee tables in front, please! Here are a few other ways to use the guest room:

❁ **Entertainment or reading room:** Add a bookcase and/or media unit to make your spare room more stimulating. Keep it organized so you don't have to straighten up when guests come to stay.

❁ **Playroom:** Use containers, along with shelves in the closet or closed cabinets, to organize toys and games. Chapter 5 provides more practical playroom tactics.

❁ **Exercise room:** If you store equipment in here, arrange places to put it away when guests come, such as crates or shelves in the closet. Big equipment such as a treadmill, rower, or bike may or may not work depending upon your space and guest traffic.

❁ **Hobby or sewing room:** A number of craft and sewing organizers are available to store hobby supplies, from model glue to beads. Fabric and patterns can go into drawers, plastic containers in the closet, or a closed wicker basket placed neatly in a corner of the room. Clean up between sessions, especially if you have small children who could get into the scissors, needles, or sewing machine.

❁ **Home office:** Save space by combining your desk and computer station into one with a specially designed piece or a desk with an extension. *Exception:* If you like to work on the computer while someone else is doing homework, a separate desk and computer table may be the way to go. For more information on a home office and household information center, see Chapter 10.

With peace permeating your personal retreats, you and your family should be resting easy. Go take a breather. There's plenty more organizing ahead!

Chapter 8

Let Me Take Your Coat!: The Entryway

First impressions count, and when it comes to your home, the front entryway creates the immediate and lasting frame of reference for everyone who walks through the door. Your guests will be delighted to arrive and take glad memories when they leave.

P-L-A-C-E the Essentials Close at Hand

Put everything in its P-L-A-C-E so that whatever the weather, you can get in and out in a snap and still leave the entryway spotless and tidy. Here's how:

❋ **Purge:** Toss or donate coats, hats, boots, and scarves that don't fit or you no longer use, unmatched or torn gloves or mittens, and any old clothes that no one claims anymore.

❋ **Like with like:** Arrange coats by owner, and sort hats, gloves, and scarves into separate groups for children and adults. For the full deal on managing the entry closet, check out Chapter 11.

❋ **Access:** Keep this season's accessories on the lower closet shelf and out-of-season items on the upper shelf. Move off-season coats to another closet or basement storage. Reserve the hall table strictly for mail and notes. Anything unrelated to leaving or entering the house can find another home.

☺ ☻ ☹ ☺ ☻ ☹ ☺ ☻ ☹ ☺ ☻ ☹ ☺ ☻ ☹ ☺ ☺ ☻ ☹ ☺

❀ **Contain:** Put hats, gloves, and scarves into clear boxes or open baskets, separating adults' from children's for quick retrieval. Hang keys on a rack near the door you use most frequently. Use baskets or a sorter on the hall table to hold incoming mail for a family.

❀ **Evaluate:** Can you easily get dressed and find everything you need to leave the house? Can you find a place for your outerwear, the mail, your keys, and what you're carrying after a long, hard day? Does the front hall stay clean with quick and easy pickups? Do you, your family, and your guests feel warmly welcomed upon walking through the front door?

Getting In and Out of the Door

The first function of the front hall is as an exit and entry. If you find yourself running around like the proverbial chicken with its head cut off when it's time to leave the house, you can put your head back on straight with a fast-start plan for using the front hall effectively.

Place everything you need by the exit door the night before. This may include the following:

❀ Briefcase, purse, backpack

❀ Keys

❀ Laptop computer

❀ Cellular phone

❀ Gym bag

❀ Tapes/CDs for the car

❀ The $10 check for your daughter's field trip

Mirror, mirror

The front hall is a great place to hang a mirror to take a last-minute look before leaving the house. In fact, feng shui practitioners hang mirrors here to aid the flow of positive energy into the house and reflect the space to make the room seem larger. Because of its prominent position, any mirror you hang in the front hall should be beautiful and in accord with your decor. If you're using a humbler model (including many full-length mirrors), consider hanging the mirror inside the closet door instead.

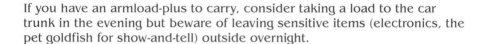
If you have an armload-plus to carry, consider taking a load to the car trunk in the evening but beware of leaving sensitive items (electronics, the pet goldfish for show-and-tell) outside overnight.

 If you leave the house by the back or garage door, place these items there for easiest access.

What goes out generally comes back in, raising the question of where all those things can go. The front hall can't be an undifferentiated dumping ground for whatever you have in your hands when you walk through the door, so think about fingertip management before you decide where to drop.

If you plan to tackle work in your briefcase or laptop computer, take the case to your work site — office, kitchen, or bedroom. Kids' backpacks can go wherever homework is done, generally the bedroom or a special spot in the kitchen (conveniently positioned to receive lunches the next morning).

 Leave by the door items that will go out with you tomorrow and you don't need in the meantime. *Exception:* Purses and wallets. Even if you live alone, your front hall can be a very public place, and keeping your cash out of temptation's way is best.

Men's wallets can go on a valet tray in the bedroom. Women can designate a spot in the bedroom to drop their purses every time they walk in the front door. Keeping your handbags in the same spot eliminates the guess-work of where you left your purse last.

Hall Table

If you have room, you may elect to put a table in the front hall. A front entry surface is likely to attract items from all who pass by, which makes the table very handy, or an organizational hell, depending on the way you use it. See Table 8-1 for a quick reference about how to optimize your hall table.

 For a power hall table that facilitates flow through the front entryway, find one with a drawer or two to hold and hide keys, sunglasses, and paper and pen for notes. Give the drawers a ruthless cleaning every week and watch this spot like a hawk.

☺ ☺ ☺ ☺ ☺ ☺ ☺ ☺ ☺ ☺ ☺ ☺ ☺ ☺ ☺ ☺ ☺ ☺ ☺ ☺

Table 8-1 Optimizing Your Front Hall Table

Good Uses for the Hall Table	Bad Uses for the Hall Table
Incoming mail area	Mail filing area
Outgoing mail drop	Return and repair center
Key depository	Anything-goes repository
Communication center for notes	

Keeping it neat and moving: The mail center

The key to good mail handling, in the hall or anywhere, is to keep it neat and moving.

❁ If you live alone, place the mail on the table when you come in.

❁ If there are two or three of you, have whoever brings in the mail sort it by recipient. You can stick to simple piles or get fancy with attractive baskets or trays.

❁ For a household of four or more, consider buying a small mail sorter.

Daily removal of mail from the front hall is a must. In fact, feel free to assign your letter carrier duties to various family members on a rotating basis. Even the youngest kids can get involved, though you probably should hand them one stack at a time and tell them the exact location to put it. Use a chart like the one in Table 8-2 to get started.

Table 8-2 Daily Mail Delivery

Family Member	Day of the Week	Completed
Mom		
Dad		

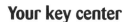

Your key center

The closest use for keys is near the door or the car, so depending on your setup, your key spot should be in the front hall or by the garage door. A drawer in the hall table or key rack on the wall provides the place; you provide the willpower to put your keys in the drawer or on the rack.

Use your head when deciding what keys to carry each day. Carry just the keys you need, which means you can leave the keys for the storage shed and your spouse's or children's cars at home. Keep the office filing cabinet keys — you guessed it — at the office.

Chapter 9

Where Dirty Is Clean Again: The Laundry or Utility Room

Air the dirty laundry: You probably spend far more time than you like in an overheated room that smells like lint in a losing battle to keep your closets stocked with clean clothes. How can you ever win?

Weary washers of the world take heart. Getting organized in the laundry room can take a big load off your mind and lighten your burden of chores.

The Cleanest Room in the P-L-A-C-E

The laundry room is a place for making things clean, so put everything into P-L-A-C-E by applying these five organizing principles:

❋ **Purge:** Toss out old laundry supplies; bent, misshapen, or excess hangers; worn or torn dust rags; and any dried-up or old craft or holiday supplies in your utility center.

❋ **Like with like:** Put laundry supplies together by type above, next to, or between the machines, right where you use them.

❋ **Access:** Keep hampers in bedroom closets to collect dirty laundry at the source. In the laundry room, create a sorting center, drying center, ironing center, and utility center to complete each task in one spot.

❋ **Contain:** Keep laundry supplies in cabinets or shelving units near the machines. Place the ironing tools in an organizer on the wall or door. Put craft supplies in clear containers and label them for easy access.

❋ **Evaluate:** Do dirty clothes easily make their way into the right load? Can you reach all the laundry supplies while standing at the machine? Can you sort clean clothes without taking a step?

☺ ☹ ☹ ☺ ☹ ☹ ☺ ☹ ☹ ☺ ☹ ☹ ☺ ☹ ☹ ☺ ☺ ☹ ☹ ☺

Doing the Laundry Where You Live

If you have a choice, locate your laundry room and your bedrooms on the same floor. But no matter where you do your laundry, you can save time and steps by keeping a hamper for dirty clothes in each bedroom, where clothes can be deposited as each person undresses.

Hallway facilities

Hallway washer-dryer setups usually accommodate just the machines and a few cabinets or shelves above. Forget about spreading out a bunch of laundry baskets. At best you can stow baskets on top of the machines while the laundry is inside; at worst — if the machines themselves are stacked — the baskets must be stored in the bedrooms at all times. You also have limited space for storing supplies, sorting, and air-drying — but read on for tips about facilitating each of these tasks.

The laundry room

A dedicated laundry room provides the space you need to get the job done with ease, *if* you arrange the room well and refrain from filling it up with other stuff.

To give everyone easy access to supplies and key areas for doing laundry, divide the laundry area into the following centers:

❀ Sorting center for dirty and clean clothes

❀ Drying center

❀ Ironing center

A well-stocked laundry room can conquer many a stain and ensure you always have the right product for the job. But a box of detergent you can't find has zero cleaning power, and shuffling through bottles when you have a big pile of dirty clothes staring you down can raise your irritation quotient fast. The right storage systems can help you whip your supplies into place and lose the laundry blues. The following can make laundry simple:

❀ **Shelves or cabinets above the machines:** A couple of midlevel shelves above your washer and dryer can contain your detergent and fabric softener at closest possible use. Solid shelving is better than wire racks because the smooth surface provides better balance to small containers and prevents any drips or leaks from oozing down behind the machines. The advantage of cabinets is that you close the doors and hide things away.

☺ ☹ ☻ ☺ ☹ ☻ ☺ ☹ ☻ ☺ ☹ ☻ ☺ ☹ ☻ ☺ ☺ ☹ ☻ ☺

❋ **Caddies next to or between machines:** From rolling wire rack shelves to slim towers that slip between the washer and dryer, there's a laundry caddy to suit every need. Look for one that works with your layout and can hold all your supplies in one place.

Group supplies by type, so that all the detergents and bleaches go together close by the washing machine with stain treatments alongside. If you treat stains in a sink or on a worktable, then put your anti-stain products near there.

Apartment laundry rooms and public Laundromats

Organizing your laundry is all the more important if your residence has no laundry facilities. Designate a spot — under the kitchen or bathroom sink; in the linen closet, utility closet, or pantry; or in a back hall — to store all your supplies and a stash of quarters. Use a rolling hamper and portable supply caddy to ease transport.

Keep at least enough quarters on hand to wash and dry all the loads you typically do in a session. Whether you buy a roll of quarters at the bank or accumulate change in a jar, you can cut out hustling for coins from your chore.

Sorting Systems

Sorting, the first step to laundry success, can be as simple or as complicated as your clothes collection requires.

A well-organized sorting system can help you rise above those piles on the floor and keep each load neat and contained. Sorting solutions on the market include a set of canvas bags hanging from a frame with a hinge-top table above for folding, sliding baskets set into a standing frame to maximize your vertical space, and the old-fashioned method of baskets set on a table.

To sort clothes the savvy way, do the following:

1 Filter out garments bound for the dry cleaners before garments go anywhere, preferably in the bedroom.

Designate a separate hamper or hanging spot in the closet for items to take to the cleaners.

2 Sort laundry loads by color.

The basic three groups are whites, darks, and mixed. Separate along these color lines and you have an excellent chance of pulling clothes from the washer representing the same spot on the spectrum as they did when they went in. Cross the lines and all bets are off.

Although the basic three categories can take care of singles, couples, and couples, and small young families, larger families and active kids can call for advanced sorting calculus that accounts for both volume — how much can fit in the machine at one time — and temperature. Leotards, shorts, and sport tops for gymnastics, cheerleading, and the health club need cold water, but all those plain white T-shirts can go gray if they don't get washed hot. If you're really down in the laundry trenches, your categories may look more like this:

Whites (no dark design): Hot

Light mixed: Warm

Dark mixed: Cold

Sheets: Hot or warm

Towels: Hot or warm

White dress shirts and blouses: Warm or cold

Dark dress shirts and blouses: Cold

Knits: Cold

Jeans: Warm

Sweat clothes: Warm or cold

Pajamas: Warm

Use Table 9-1 to create your own laundry sorting chart. Post it in the laundry room where everyone can see it (and sort!).

Table 9-1 Your Family's Sorting Guide

Load	Temperature	Favorite Detergent

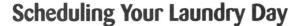

Scheduling Your Laundry Day

Accustomed to doing laundry when you run out of clothes? There is a better way. You can schedule your wash in one of two ways: all on one day, or split into two. If you work every day, you may want to leave weekends free for errands, outings, and fun, in which case splitting up the job into one weeknight for linens and another for clothes would be best. On the other hand, if you have a young family, you may prefer to get the whole thing out of the way on Saturday or Sunday, when your spouse or a babysitter can take the kids or a play date can be arranged. Either way, if you find yourself frequently staring at an empty closet, your schedule needs refining.

Utility or Mudroom

The laundry room often doubles as a mudroom off the back or basement door, where everything from sandy beach towels to crusty boots can congregate. Your utility room may serve as an extra storage spot, or a place to do anything messy. The more hats your laundry room wears, the more you need to organize.

The mess-free mudroom

Though you may not think of the mudroom as wearing a public face, this is a primary point of entry to the house, and family and guests alike may troop through after swimming, picnicking, or playing. Make it nice and easy:

❋ Add a closed cabinet for beach towels, bath towels, and supplies if you have a shower and/or bathroom here. (See Chapter 6 for more on setting up a beautiful and functional bath area.)

❋ Use a closed cabinet or shoe rack for sports shoes and organize them by owner.

❋ Keep sports clothes neat with designated hanging space, baskets on shelves, or a standalone cabinet.

❋ Relocate sports equipment to the garage for easiest access.

Utility unlimited

Utility means "useful," which often translates as storage. If you have more space than you need to get the wash done, consider these additional storage uses for the laundry room:

☺ ☻ ☹ ☺ ☻ ☹ ☺ ☻ ☹ ☺ ☻ ☹ ☺ ☻ ☹ ☺ ☺ ☻ ☹ ☺

❋ **Extra refrigerator and/or freezer.**

❋ **Holiday serving pieces and supplies.**

❋ **Hobby and craft supplies.** If you don't have a dedicated area and usually do your work close by — for instance, if the laundry room is on the first floor and you stage your craft sessions in the kitchen — then store crafts here.

Cleaning up the laundry room can leave you better dressed and less stressed. Don't get sidelined by stains or worried by wrinkles. Get organized!

Chapter **10**

PCs, Printers, and Paper Clips: The Home Office

In This Chapter

☺ Setting up your home office

☺ Organizing the right tools for the job

☺ Using technology to keep your workflow flowing

Your home office may be your primary workplace, or just a site for handling work you brought home from headquarters. In either case, making your home workplace work can provide professional results from everything you do there.

A basic principle for any workplace is that you want to minimize distractions. At home, you have to balance that priority with available space and your own personal style. Ask yourself a few questions to get started:

✿ How much space do you need to accomplish your tasks and store your supplies? (The layout process should provide the answer to this.)

✿ Do you prefer solitude and quiet, or do you need to know what's going on in the rest of the house?

✿ What temperature and lighting conditions make you most productive? Where can they be found?

Choosing a Location for Your Home Office

The best solution is a dedicated room. Second best is an infrequently used room, such as a guest bedroom, that can be devoted to business 90 percent of the time. Last on the list, but sometimes the only alternative, is sharing space with a family/media room, kitchen, or bedroom. Don't worry. You can make the available room work!

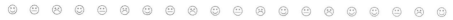
Choose the best location for your home office by referring to the pros and cons listed in Table 10-1.

If your home office must share space with another function, create a visual and psychological divider with a tall bookcase or decorative tri-fold screen.

Table 10-1 Home Office Locations

Place	Pros	Cons
Basement	Quiet and isolated for working and thinking	Can be windowless, dark, and cold. You don't know whether the weather is right for a run to the office store or copy place, or if the kids are home from school.
Guest bedroom	All yours when guests aren't there. Most of the closet is free for storing supplies.	No work possible when you have guests. Need to compete for space with bedroom furniture, which may tempt you to catch a few zzz's when you should be working.
Media room	Great double use of space for singles	Other household members are likely to be blasting music or movies.
Bedroom	Many apartment and condo dwellers have no choice. Leaves living room uncluttered and restful.	Hard to sleep peacefully in your office with your desk staring you down. Your partner's sleep schedule may be interrupted. Space is limited.
Kitchen	Allows you to get to basic household paperwork while still watching the kids and staying in the thick of things.	Constant distractions on this stretch of household superhighway. Forget about making client calls from here. Watch out for curious hands.

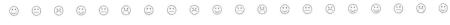

Peak Productivity Placement

Now is the time to put everything into place. Your goal? Fingertip management of everything you do. The way to get there? Blueprint your workspace. You may not be an architect, but anyone can benefit from drawing up a floor plan to find the most productive office placement. You may discover a new way to face your desk for better concentration, hidden space for another file cabinet, or a nifty arrangement to put all your reference books within reach.

Drawing up the blueprint

Refer back to the section on blueprint basics in Chapter 2, and follow the instructions to draw your office to scale, mark the windows and doors, and create furniture cutouts. Add cutouts in a different color to represent equipment.

Start playing with P-L-A-C-E-ment of your cutouts on your floor plan to come up with one or more schemes that put each task within easy reach:

❀ **Purge:** Get rid of all unused or ill-suited furniture and equipment. You can donate distracting artwork to a charity or put it elsewhere.

❀ **Like with like:** Line up your file cabinets. Find one spot for all your books. Create work centers for different activities by grouping together everything you need for a task.

❀ **Access:** Arrange your workspace by placing furniture and equipment in a parallel, L-shape, or U-shape layout for better fingertip management. Check out Figure 10-1 for examples of each layout. Parallel layouts provide a space-efficient floor plan for jobs requiring a limited number of references and resources. An L-shaped layout, offers a little more privacy in a semi-enclosed space. While the U-shaped configuration puts the most resources within reach.

❀ **Contain:** Put files into file cabinets and books into bookcases or credenzas. Under-desk drawers can keep supplies off the counter-top. Finally, make sure you have a way to contain everything — for instance, add a credenza for the books and binders currently stacked on top of your workstation.

❀ **Evaluate:** How do you feel when you walk into your office? How does your flow go in the thick of a project or stressful situation? Can you balance the checkbook, check your e-mail, and finish your neighborhood newsletter without leaving your chair?

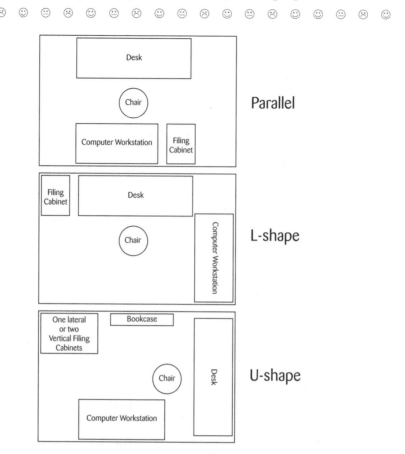

Figure 10-1: Workspace layouts that put tools at your fingertips.

Using space effectively

Use the space beneath windows by placing a desk, short bookcase, or two-drawer file cabinet there. This is not the spot for a standard bookcase, a four-drawer file cabinet, or a tall computer workstation, unless you want to lose your view.

Move the desk out toward the center of the room to slip a credenza, bookcase, or file cabinet behind it. Take a ruler and measure your files from front to back to assess how many inches of storage space you need. Allow room (1 to 2 inches) for growth. You should also allow clearance to pull out file cabinet drawers to double the cabinet's depth. Typical file cabinet dimensions are:

❀ **Vertical:** 15 inches (letter) or 18 inches (legal) wide by 21 inches to 36 inches deep.

❀ **Lateral:** 36 inches (letter) or 42 inches (legal) wide by 18 inches deep.

Furniture: The basics

What do you need to furnish your space for good work? Use the following discussions to start your list, marking what you have, what you want, and what you don't need.

Finding the right desk

The right desk provides just enough surface area to get all your jobs done (more would be a waste of room space) and a layout that allows fingertip management of each task. Assess your needs in these two dimensions and choose between three desk formats:

❀ **Standard:** This is your basic rectangle, a space-efficient bet if you don't use a computer at your desk or have a separate computer workstation.

❀ **L-shaped:** Add a perpendicular piece to a regular desk and you have an L shape, with the second side just right to hold a computer, to spread out papers 11 x 17 or larger, or to collate materials.

❀ **U-shaped:** Adding a third side to the desk allows you to easily toggle between a regular desktop, a computer station, and a clear space for big projects. You can also create a U shape with your layout as described earlier in the chapter, which, depending on your needs, may be a better way.

No matter what shape desk you choose, look for two to four small drawers and one to two file drawers to keep everything in fingertip reach.

Choosing your computer workstation

When choosing a computer workstation, whether as part of a desk or a standalone unit, measure all your components — monitor, CPU tower, speakers, printer, scanner — then look for:

❀ Enough surface area to hold what you need on the desktop. This definitely includes your monitor and enough space to open up files, books, and reports to work from. You may also need room for a keyboard, printer, speakers, and disk holder.

97

❀ A pullout drawer to get the keyboard off the desktop.

❀ A drawer for pens and pencils.

❀ Shelves for reference books and/or disk trays.

❀ Another shelf for your printer or speakers. You can also use a pull-out drawer in a cabinet below to hold the printer.

❀ A built-in disk holder if you need a lot of disks on hand.

❀ Floor space or a shelf for the CPU. Skip the closed cabinet, which is one more door to open every time you want to swap disks or reboot.

Other office essentials

A good ergonomic office chair with wheels will make your life easier and your back happier. Put a plastic mat on the floor for smooth rolling from the desk to the computer, credenza, bookcase, or file cabinet.

A table and mini-bookshelf in one, a credenza can clear off your desk by holding the books or binders you need every day inside. Put a telephone, fax machine, printer, or small copier on top to get double-duty from the piece and prevent piles of paper from forming there.

If your work requires many reference materials — you're a lawyer, human resources administrator, professor, or writer — then a bookcase with adjustable shelves is the way to get those stacks of books off the floor. Organize your library by subject matter as described in Chapter 4.

 Stop! Before you buy a single file cabinet, skip to Chapter 14 and follow the file-purging instructions. See how your space and budget requirements downsize?

Next consider whether you should contain files in lateral or vertical cabinets. Vertical file cabinets, which pull out so the files are facing you, extend farther into the room in both closed and open position. Lateral cabinets, in which the files are perpendicular to you as you pull out the drawer, stick out less but take up more wall space. You may need to do your layout, as explained later in this chapter, before you make your decision.

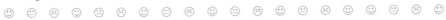

Clearing the desktop

Try this simple system for clearing off the desk and setting up all your accessories and supplies for fingertip management of your job:

❀ **Clear the desktop of anything that catches your eye such as in/out boxes, papers and files, photos, or knickknacks.** Clear off photos by hanging them on the wall behind you or finding a display spot off your desk and outside your direct line of vision. Snowplow piles by using the right-now rule: If you're not using the paper or file right now, put it away.

❀ **Remove items that you don't use every day.** Consider sticky notes, the memo pad, staple remover, paper clips, binder clips, rubber bands, tape, scissors, ruler, highlighter, markers, calculator, and disk tray, and put away those that don't pass the everyday test. Staplers and calculators are questionable contenders. If they get daily use, you can keep them on the desk, but if they don't and you have room in a drawer, off they go. See Table 10-2 for an everyday use checklist.

❀ **For fingertip management, put everything you reach for on your preferred side: the hand you write with.** Relocate pens, pencils, notepad, calculator, and disk tray to your writing side. The telephone is the big exception to the rule. Pick up the receiver with your preferred hand and you'll see why: With your writing hand busy, you can't take notes. Switching to the other ear leaves you with a phone cord strapped across your chest (or around your neck on really bad days). Move the phone to the opposite side.

❀ **Create mini-desktop work centers for the phone, computer, and clock.** The telephone center includes the phone, a message pad or log alongside, and the address and phone index slightly farther back. If you have an answering machine, that would be the item farthest to the back. Put disks next to your monitor to form a computer center, and group your calendar and clock to create a time center.

To help smooth your way through this process, use Table 10-2 to help you decide what to keep on top of your desk. Things you use several times a day are the best qualified. Everyday items may be better in a drawer, and anything you use less than once a day definitely moves. Check off the appropriate column for each item, and then use the list to relocate excess desktop items.

☺ ☻ ☹ ☺ ☺ ☹ ☺ ☺ ☹ ☺ ☺ ☹ ☺ ☺ ☹ ☺ ☺ ☺ ☹ ☺

If your drawers are too crowded to receive everything you try to get off the desktop, just put it aside onto a file cabinet or shelf for now and read on.

Table 10-2 Desktop Decisions

Item	Use Every Day?	Several Times a Day?
Calendar/planner/organizer		
Pen and pencil holder		
Sticky notes		
Memo pad		
Phone message pad		
Stapler		
Staple remover		
Paper clips		
Binder clips		
Rubber bands		
Tape		
Scissors		
Ruler		
Highlighter		
Markers		
Calculator		
Disk tray		

Downsizing your desk supplies

People can get a little giddy when it comes to office supplies, like on your first day of school when you can't have enough freshly sharpened pencils. But your desk is not a supply cabinet, so start by storing all duplicate items in your closet or in a cabinet. Now take a load off your desk by sending the following stuff to the trash:

❋ Dried out pens, markers, and highlighters

❋ Stubby little pencils

❋ Dried out correction fluid

❋ Dried out glue sticks

☺ ☺ ☹ ☺ ☺ ☹ ☺ ☺ ☹ ☺ ☺ ☹ ☺ ☺ ☹ ☺ ☺ ☺ ☹ ☹ ☺

❀ Stretched out rubber bands and paper clips

❀ Small sections of staples that jam the stapler

❀ Promotional items you don't use

Restock a supply just comfortably before you run out. When you load the last strip of staples into the stapler, that's the time to pick up the next box.

Arranging Your Work Centers

A mess at your computer workstation can create such a mess in your mind that no amount of electronic intelligence can compensate. Use organizing principles to keep everything in its place as you work at the computer, and you can take full advantage of technology's awesome power.

Divvying up drawers

Group like things together: staples and tape, mail supplies, and so forth. Next, achieve fingertip management by putting the things you often need access to in the drawer closest to you. Contain items with drawer dividers so everything stays in place.

If you have no desk drawers — perhaps you're working at an old kitchen table — several options are available to remedy the situation:

❀ **A pullout drawer that attaches under the desktop.**

❀ **A desktop drawer set.** Get creative by placing the drawers on a file cabinet or credenza to keep your desktop clear.

❀ **A rolling cart of drawers.**

❀ **A two-drawer file cabinet under the desk or within reach behind or to the side of you.**

Now turn each of your drawers into a work center:

❀ **The central drawer is the pen/pencil center:** pens, pencils, ruler, scissors, markers, clips, tape, correction fluid, staples, staple remover, and so on.

❀ **The top small drawer becomes a mail and filing center:** stamps, address labels, envelopes, business cards, hanging file tabs, file labels, and blank address cards.

❀ **The second small drawer turns into a stationery/paper center:** letterhead, stationery, and notepads.

❀ **The file drawer is the project center:** "take action" file and current major project files.

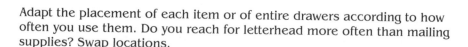
Adapt the placement of each item or of entire drawers according to how often you use them. Do you reach for letterhead more often than mailing supplies? Swap locations.

With your drawer floor plan in place, the time to divvy up the space is upon you. Drawer divider options include

❀ **A sectioned flat tray,** usually designed to fit the pen and pencil drawer.

❀ **A deep drawer organizer,** which is the same as the flat tray but with higher sides for a deeper drawer. This is great for tall items, such as correction fluid, or if you're short on space and need to stack — paper clips on top of a box of staples, and so on.

❀ **Separate rectangular containers** — narrow for pens and pencils, wider for other supplies.

❀ **Built-in, movable vertical dividers.** If your drawers don't include some, you can buy your own.

 Sturdy cardboard boxes and tops work just fine as drawer dividers. Try the top of a business card box to hold rubber bands.

Organizing your computer area

If you have a computer workstation, reserve the area strictly for computer supplies and keep everything else at your desk. If your desk serves double-duty, allocate computer supplies among your desktop, drawers, and/or bookshelves by grouping like items together and placing them for easy access.

P-L-A-C-E is good news to computer users suffering from disk disorder. Rather than rummaging through CDs, diskettes, manuals, and DVDs trying to find something you know you have in there somewhere, set up a system for keeping them all organized once and for all. You not only save yourself time finding what you need; you also save yourself the stress of wondering whether you lost an electronic file. Here's how to make sense of your computer media:

❀ **Purge:** Remove all computer disks that you no longer need. If you have backups of your college checking account that you closed five years ago, get rid of them. Toss or recycle the disk.

❀ **Like with like:** Use the color of disks and/or labels to categorize your media — maybe graphics disks are yellow and budget are green, or school files go on blue and business on red. If you have more than one booklet for any piece of hardware or software — printer, scanner, programs — group them together in a resealable plastic bag.

❋ **Access:** Keep your most active disks, backups, and program disks you use regularly, closest at hand. Old backups, programs you're not using, and installed programs you don't need to support by disk can be stored somewhere else, which may be off the workstation if space is tight.

❋ **Contain:** All disks can go into holders, with dividers or separate trays to distinguish between different types. Start by separating programs from backups, and then arrange by the categories established in the previous step. You can get a multimedia tray to keep different formats (floppy, CD, Zip, and so on) together.

❋ **Evaluate:** Are you keeping too many disks? Would color help you distinguish graphics from word processing or spreadsheet documents, or quickly spot client files or research information?

Why should I bother to get a computer?

If you haven't taken the plunge and purchased a home computer yet, you may not see the need. Here's a list of some ways to use a computer to save time and stay organized that just may change your mind:

❀ Store and organize phone numbers and addresses in a database. Let your modem do the dialing and your printer do the labeling!

❀ Manage your time with calendar programs that offer daily to-do lists and meeting alarms.

❀ Manage personal finances, including balancing your budget, writing checks, and exporting the data to a tax program at year's end.

❀ Do your taxes and file your tax returns electronically with programs suited to the job.

❀ Create grocery and other shopping lists in a word processing program.

❀ Make your own greeting cards with a graphics or photo program.

❀ Publish a newsletter, flyer, or announcement, complete with pro layout and graphics, with a desktop publishing program. Send it directly by e-mail if you like.

❀ Archive photos and home movies on CD, DVD, or the Internet. Many sites allow you to give friends and family a code to view them. Use programs from word processing to graphics to specialized photo- and video-editing applications to place, play with, and touch up your photos and movies in a variety of formats.

❀ Store, organize, and analyze your recipes with culinary programs, or toss all the old ones and search the Web for new recipes when you're ready to cook.

Maximizing Wired Efficiency

The type of your wired connections is becoming an increasingly important component of time management at home. *Bandwidth* is what tech-savvy people call the capacity of a line to transmit and receive data. Generally, the bigger the bandwidth of a line, the faster and more reliably information flows through it.

Divide communication lines by the way that you use them. At home, the wires you need may include

❀ Separate phone lines for business and personal use

❀ One to two more lines for fax and Internet use

❀ A separate kids' line if you have some good talkers in the family

 Before you get a second phone line for Internet use, consider other high-speed options. Many companies offer inexpensive high-speed Internet connections (like DSL, cable, or wireless satellite). Often the cost of the service is cheaper than getting a second phone line. Plus, with more bandwidth, you have the bonus of increased download/upload speed compared to a standard dial-up connection, faster page loading, and overall better performance from the Internet. If you spend lots of time online, it can really improve your productivity and save you money. Call your telephone company and/or cable or satellite TV provider to find out about services available in your area.

Paper or Electronic: A File Is a File

Whether the file comes to you by snail mail or e-mail, pops out of your printer, or sits on your hard drive, a file is a file, and you need to evaluate it and organize it accordingly. Following is a rundown of information-flow principles as they pertain to electronic files.

 You can archive computer files much more space-efficiently than paper files — so when in doubt about whether to save something, simply move the file off your hard drive and onto a backup. Place the backup date on the disk label, and send anything you haven't used in a year to the trash.

Filtering file flow: Deciding what to save

Your decision whether to save or delete a file can help keep useful information at your fingertips or drag you and your computer down with stuff you don't need. To avoid the latter scenario, you need to filter information by asking yourself some essential questions about the file in question.

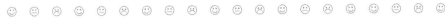
Apply the five W-A-S-T-E questions from Chapter 2 to every computer file you save, and stay as clear electronically as you aim to be in the hard-copy world:

❀ **Is it worthwhile?** Keep an e-mail from someone asking you to take on a work project and telling you how much the project pays. Toss an Internet joke. If you're going to forward it, do so right away and delete it before closing.

❀ **Will I use the file again?** Keep a handout for a presentation you may give again. Toss e-mail you answered. Note any follow-ups in your "take action" file; move the mail to the appropriate folder if you need it for official records.

❀ **Can I easily find it somewhere else?** Keep all essential computer documentation. Toss Web site printouts. Bookmark the site so you can easily find it again.

❀ **Will anything happen if I toss the file?** Keep the master school calendar, but toss the weekly reminders of holidays for the week.

❀ **Do I need the entire item?** Keep e-mails with important information or documentation. Toss unnecessary information from e-mails, like repeated information in forwards and replies.

Finalizing your electronic files

Great! You filtered the files by using W-A-S-T-E and you have a few that passed the criteria that you really do need to save. Now what? Think ABC:

❀ **Active: Distinguish between active and inactive files.** Use the criteria discussed in Chapter 14 to determine which of your electronic files are active. You can move inactive files to a backup medium or purged.

❀ **Basic: Know your basic tools.** The computer provides wonderful organizing tools in the form of filing systems you can manage with a click of the mouse: Explorer in Windows, the desktop for Mac users, and filing cabinets in many e-mail programs. In each of these, you can create folders and subfolders and use them just as you do hanging and file folders in your paper system.

❀ **Classify.** Follow the system in Chapter 14 to classify your electronic files, creating level-one folders for main categories and subfolders inside to hold subcategories. Need to go to level three for a sub-subcategory? No problem. A computer loves a classification structure that works like an index.

Just as you file papers according to category rather than how they were produced, arrange your electronic files by subject regardless of what program they come from. Centralizing by subject makes it easier to find and

105

☺ ☹ ☺ ☺ ☹ ☺ ☺ ☹ ☺ ☺ ☹ ☺ ☺ ☹ ☺ ☺ ☹ ☺

open everything you need in order to work on a project, as well as to back up new information at the end of the day.

Unfortunately, computers don't currently provide a way to use color in your filing system. However, color is a great tool in word processing and other documents, where you can use colored type or highlighting to call attention to key areas, edits, or questions.

Part 3

Organizing Storage Spaces

You may think you're organized because you have separate storage spaces. But what are you keeping in those spaces? How long have they been there? Do you need them? What's the cost of pitching them? The cost of keeping them? This part helps you answer those questions.

The chapters in this part can help you put everything away in secret spaces, so *storage* is no longer synonymous with *stress*. You may even discover that storing more is sometimes less. So get busy in the basement! Get going in the garage! If you follow these guidelines, you may even have room for the car.

Chapter 11

No Safe Haven for Junk: Tackling Closets

Closets may be the single most used organizing tool in the American household. Not only does just about everyone have at least one, but they also include this handy door that closes, so you don't have to look at all the junk you've shoved in it. This chapter gives you details for making every closet in your home a paradigm of efficiency and a true partner in getting your house in order.

The Bedroom Closet

Take a deep breath. This may hurt a little bit, but the reward is that you'll finally open your closet door without fear and realize your wardrobe's full potential. Clean up your clothes with six steps that will change the way you dress for the better:

1 **Fashion changes each year, so go through every item in your closet, from shoes to suits and everything in between, and purge anything you haven't worn in the last 12 months or won't be able to squeeze into soon.**

   This is a great opportunity to figure out what flatters you and jettison the deadweight.

2 **Move your off-season duds offsite.**

   Even if you live in a warm climate, you probably have at least a spring/summer and fall/winter wardrobe. Relocate your off-season clothes to a closet in the guest bedroom, attic, or basement, or into storage-area boxes.

3   Double tier or layer.

If you have one closet rod and many short garments such as shirts, blouses, jackets, and skirts, adding a second rod underneath can double your storage space. Home improvement people can install rod number two directly into closet walls; those less inclined can opt for an add-a-rod that simply hangs from the one you have. Layering is another space expander if you have a long-hanging area. Here you hang a bar with holes for additional hangers from the rod. Keep a single color of garment on a bar so that you know just where to look for what. For the kids' closet, it may be useful to start with two groups — school and play — and then subdivide from there. Consult Figure 11-1 to see how easy double-tiering or layering can be.

4   Organize like with like; think occasion first, and then type of garment.

Dressing for work is always a time-sensitive affair, so if you work out-side the home, put all your professional clothes in the place most accessible when you open the door. You can delve deeper for casual clothes, when you have more time. If you're sharing a closet and have two double-tiered sections, each person takes one for short clothes and the rest of the closet can be split between the two. If there's only one tiered section, the taller person gets the higher rod. Devote this section to shirts — dress, and then casual. Within your work and casual categories, divide by garment type and then style.

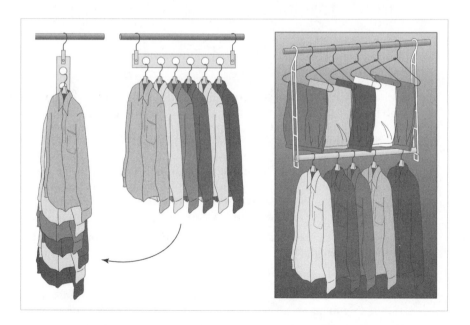

Figure 11-1: An adjustable second rod doubles closet space in a snap.

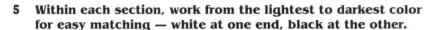

5 **Within each section, work from the lightest to darkest color for easy matching — white at one end, black at the other.**

Exception: Putting navy blue and black together invites chromatic confusion, so separate these two colors with the red/pink family, or put multicolored garments in between them.

6 **Stock the shelves.**

If you have a walk-in closet short on shelves with room to spare, build them in! The ideal candidates for shelf space are sweaters, T-shirts, shoes, purses, scarves, hats, and extra blankets or pillows. In kids' rooms, use them to store toys and games for little kids, and then sweaters as the children grow up. Don't build shelves into a small closet, though; using free-standing shelves or a chest of drawers that can be removed as a child's clothes-hanging requirements grow is better. High, hard-to-reach shelves are a good place to store off-season items, such as blankets and sweaters during the summer. Clamp dividers onto top shelves to section them off and keep things from falling over.

Calling all fashionistas: Shoes

The best shoe organizer for you is the one that works with your shoes and your space. Here are a few tips:

❁ If you have a free wall, use stackable units for vertical height. Wooden shelving is great because it has flat surfaces for heels or flats. The metal units often require hanging heels over the back and so take a little more effort and time.

❁ Open wooden cubes — still stackable; still work.

❁ A hanging rack or pockets on the back of the closet door can do the trick if you don't have sliding doors or more than a door's worth of shoes. Pockets don't hold heels well, though — they stick out at you like weapons.

No matter what storage system you use, arrange your shoes as you do your clothes: by color and moving from light to dark. (Sorting shoes by style is tricky, so stick to color to keep things simple.)

Assembling accessories

Fashion experts tell us that accessories make the outfit. Unfortunately, the things that top off an outfit really tangle up the closet. Here's how to contain them and relieve accessory angst:

- ❀ **Ties and belts:** Racks are the rule for sorting out belts and ties, and you can find them in formats from flat to revolving.

- ❀ **Scarves:** If you have a free drawer or shelf, fold your scarves and lay them flat, layered ¼ inch apart so you can see the edge of each one. Angle the fold toward you so it's easy to pull.

- ❀ **Purses:** Start by considering: Do you really need more than a black, brown, navy, white, and dress purse? If so, store off-season purses as you do clothes and sort the rest by color. Arrange them on a shelf in the closet with their straps tucked in to avoid tangles.

- ❀ **Caps:** If you have just a few caps, put some self-adhesive hooks inside the closet door and hang them there. For a larger cap collection, buy a high-capacity rack to hang in your front or bedroom closet.

The Coat Closet

If you have a standard-issue front hall closet — one rod and one shelf — the first thing to do is add another shelf. Front closets usually have plenty of extra space above, and if need be you can usually lower the rod a little to make space for the second shelf.

Next, think one-stop centers in setting up the closet, dividing items by like type and owner, and arranging them for easy access.

Family coat center

Human nature encourages people to hang their coats in the hall closet any which way, which doesn't work very well. Group coats by the identity of their owner so that whoever opens the closet door can easily match his choice to the occasion, the outfit, and the conditions outside. Start with the adults' coats on the end of the closet closest to the doorknob and work your way down to the youngest child closest to the hinge.

 You may be tempted to economize on space by installing an extra closet rod closer to the floor for shorter children's jackets. Bright idea, but the additional rod doesn't work so well in this closet. Children grow up quickly and get longer coats. In the meantime, grown-ups and guests need a place to stow their full-length wraps without short rods in the way.

Accessory center

Many households accumulate acres of accessories and few have devised an optimal system for storing and accessing mittens, gloves, earmuffs, scarves, sun hats, ski caps, or the dog's leash. Here's how to solve your own accessory overload:

1 **Purge unmatched gloves and mittens, worn or torn items, and anything no one's worn in a year.**

2 **Sort your gear into winter and summer groups.**

   Put rain-related stuff with the current season because rain can fall in either half of the year.

3 **Organize each seasonal group by putting like items together: gloves, hats, scarves, and so forth.**

   Separate kids' stuff from the adults'. If your family is really big and you have space, make a separate stack for each child.

4 **Contain each group in its own colored basket.**

   For instance, you could put adult gloves in blue, kids' gloves in green, and so on. If you'd rather see contents than basket color, opt for clear containers instead. Label the baskets or containers.

5 **Access what you need now by placing the out-of-season containers on the closet's upper shelf, and then arranging this season's accessories on the easy-to-reach lower shelf.**

Umbrellas can stand in a corner of the closet, or you can use the handle or loop to hang them on a closet wall hook, over a hanger, or (for the hook-style handles) over the closet rod. If you're in a rainy spot or season, a stand by the door can receive wet umbrellas; relocate the whole thing to the garage or basement during sunny months.

Closet of All Trades: The Linen Closet

Whether your linen closet is in the bathroom or the hall outside, you should always be able to open the door and easily pull out a clean set of sheets or towels. This is also the place to look for backups of toilet paper or soap. And what a handy spot for a hammer, the shoe polish, the upstairs cleaning supplies. Everything is possible when you put everything in its place, as follows:

✸ **Pull everything out of your linen closet and toss or donate the excess baggage, including threadbare, stained, and unmatched sheets and towels.** One extra set of sheets per bed, plus a set sized for a sofa bed if you have one will do. A total of two towel sets per person is plenty for basic household needs. Add up to two sets for guests, four hand towels per guest bathroom, and a beach towel for each family member (four more if guests swim at your house).

☺ ☹ ☹ ☺ ☹ ☹ ☺ ☹ ☹ ☺ ☹ ☹ ☺ ☹ ☹ ☺ ☹ ☹ ☺

❋ **Select the items that are best stored in the linen closet and group them by like type for easy access.**

❋ **Think high-low.** Store items that are seldom used or dangerous to children on the highest shelves, small things that are hard to spot at eye level, and light but big items below. For higher-middle shelves, think personal-care items, first-aid kit, shoe care, cleaning supplies, and toolbox. The middle-lower shelves can be used for bed and bath linens while the bottom shelves or floor can accommodate bath and facial tissue, extra blankets, trash bags, travel cosmetic/ shaving kits, and a sick bucket.

❋ **Group and stack.** If jamming your clean sheets onto the shelf is something like pushing your way onto a New York subway car, it's time to clean up your act. The right folding technique can stack your sheets up neatly with an easy visual ID of what's what. Next are personal-care items and cleaning supplies: Contain items in clear or different colored baskets, grouped by like type, and make it easy (or difficult for kids) to access what you need. Pullout drawers that sit on the shelf can help. Add labels so that one look takes you to your target.

Chapter 12

Upstairs, Downstairs: The Basement and Attic

Why do people love to hate their basements and attics? Because they give folks a place to stash their secret messes and in the process can cause a cycle of guilt that grows with the piles. My recommendation to every client is to give these out-of-sight spaces a position front and center in your organized mind.

Even if you lack a basement or attic, read on for strategies that can be adapted to any area of the house.

The P-L-A-C-E for Storage

Clutter doesn't stop clogging up your life just because you don't look at the mess every day. In fact, for some people hidden clutter is the biggest burden of all. So tackle your basement and attic with P-L-A-C-E and get more value from your real estate.

❀ **Purge:** Toss out any broken, torn, and worn items as well as return/repair items that have been out of use for a year or more. Duplicate tools; dried out glue, paint, and varnish; and old or excess workshop and hobby supplies get the heave-ho, too.

❀ **Like with like:** Arrange all storage items by type — off-season clothing, entertaining supplies, rotating toys, and so on.

☺ ☻ ☹ ☺ ☻ ☹ ☺ ☻ ☹ ☺ ☻ ☹ ☺ ☻ ☹ ☺ ☺ ☻ ☹ ☺

❋ **Access:** Establish storage, workshop, hobby/craft, exercise, and gift-wrap centers. Keep flammable items away from the furnace and hot-water heater.

❋ **Contain:** Keep large tools on a pegboard and parts in mini-drawers. Hobby and craft supplies can go in divided drawers or cabinets (possibly childproof). Exercise equipment may be contained nicely in boxes, while gift-wrap supplies can go into plastic containers.

❋ **Evaluate:** Can you find storage items in a flash? Do you look forward to working in your workshop or hobby area? Can you easily exercise whenever the energy strikes? Are young children safe from dangerous equipment, tools, and supplies?

Down in the Depths: Functional Concerns

In the basement, clutter around equipment and machinery is inconvenient when you need service and dangerous if the jumble is flammable. A disorganized storage area makes finding and getting to items stored there difficult, sometimes impossible, so what's the point of holding onto them, anyway? A mess won't motivate anyone to get busy in the workshop or exercise center. And the whole thing can turn into a swamp of ruined stuff if a seemingly simple shower turns into a flood while you're at work or out to dinner and you're unprepared. The basement and its functions essentially boil down to three basic needs:

❋ A holding place for appliances that run the house — furnace, water heater, water softener, and so forth

❋ Storage

❋ Places for activity centers such as the laundry room, workshop, hobby or craft shop, exercise area, playroom, or family room

The most important thing to do in the basement is to store all chemicals and valuable items on shelves or tables above flood level. Even if you don't live near water and no threat of serious flooding is present in your geographic location, water from especially heavy rain can make your basement a mud basin and a safety hazard. Being organized beforehand can lessen the degree of any such disaster.

Here are some additional precautions to keep the basement functional and friendly.

❋ **Clear out the space around the furnace, water heater, other major appliances, pipes, and drains.** Be particularly mindful of flammable and heat-sensitive items, as well as any valuables that

☺ ☺ ☹ ☺ ☺ ☹ ☺ ☺ ☹ ☺ ☺ ☹ ☺ ☺ ☹ ☺ ☺ ☺ ☹ ☺

may suffer beneath a burst pipe. Section off this area with a locked door if you have small children. To keep from fumbling for keys in the event of an emergency, a simple hook too high for a child to reach can do the job.

❋ **Install a sump pump to fight floods.**

❋ **Install another sump pump — this one battery-operated for backup during power failures.**

❋ **Keep a large, battery-powered flashlight on hand to check equipment and the fuse box if the power fails.**

❋ **Maintain critical equipment on a regular basis.** Set up a schedule and post it on the wall use Table12-1 for a starting point. Check out *The Parent's Success Guide to Managing a Household* (published by Wiley) for maintenance tips.

 Don't risk turning your basement into toxic soup by storing chemicals — for cleaning, garden care, household jobs, or hobbies — where floodwaters can reach them.

Table 12-1 Maintenance Checklist

Equipment	Maintenance	Date	Next Scheduled

Storage Made Simple

Whether in the basement, the attic, or anywhere at all, storage can and should be simple, but many people miss the boat by storing things willy-nilly and without a plan. The complicated results tax the mind and make retrieving things difficult, which defeats the purpose of storing them to begin with. There are two steps to simple storage: Decide what to keep, and then figure out where and how to keep it. W-A-S-T-E and P-L-A-C-E break these big questions down into bite-sized decisions.

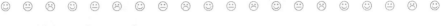

Deciding what to keep

The five W-A-S-T-E questions (see Chapter 2) can help you zero in on what's worth keeping, and what's a waste of space and the time you spend dealing with it. Put each item to the W-A-S-T-E test before you put it into the box or onto the shelf.

* **Worthwhile?** Do I ever use this? Do I really need it? What if I just took a photo and filed it under "Memories"? Items that you really want or need are probably worth storing, while those that are expendable or you haven't used in several years fail this test and should be tossed or donated.

* **Again?** Will I actually use this item again, or am I keeping it in case of some unlikely future or because I paid good money for it? Sure, this made a great decoration for my son's first birthday party but now he's in grade school and the moment's long gone. No matter how valuable something was to you in the past, if you won't use the item again, don't waste the storage space. Discard.

* **Somewhere else?** How many spare hair dryers does a family really need? Couldn't I borrow my neighbor's pasta machine if I ever have that authentic Italian dinner party I've been thinking about for five years? If you can easily find an item somewhere else if and when the need arises, whether by borrowing or even buying a new one, don't store. Say goodbye instead.

* **Toss it?** Will my life change for the worse without my box of high-school papers on hand? What happens if I haul this dusty old broken-down chair to the dumpster? If you can imagine tossing an item without clear negative consequences, go ahead and do so.

* **Entire item?** Do you need the full set of luggage, or do you only use the carry-on? If you love the punch bowl but always serve in paper cups, why take up storage space with the unused cup set? Just because something came in a set doesn't mean you need to store every piece. Sort out the useful parts or pieces and throw or give away the rest.

Now that you ran the gauntlet, let me assure you that there's nothing wrong with storing things. Storing is an organizational basic: If you don't use something every day, storage is the way to keep it out of the way.

 You can whip things in and out of storage more quickly if you can see what you're doing, so install enough lights to illuminate every nook and cranny of your storage area.

Where and how to keep it: Basic storage principles

Though you use storage items less frequently than other things, some principles of P-L-A-C-E are still the guide for putting them away.

Like with like saves the day. Group all your storage items by category. Think like a calendar when organizing holiday items, devoting a separate container to each major celebration and arranging them chronologically. Smaller holidays for which you store less stuff — Valentine's Day, Fourth of July, and so on — can be grouped together.

Store things close to where you use them, saving prime spots to access the most-frequently used items. For instance, if you break out your big coffee-maker every time company comes, keep it near the front of your storage area, but once-a-year holiday supplies can go farther back. If the basement has a door out to the garage, store sports equipment as close to the door as you can. Save the corner of the shelf closest to your work center to keep extra craft supplies.

Containing items makes them easier to group, find, move, and stack, and also keeps them out of the dust. You have various enclosure options, each with its own best use:

* **Cases:** When items come already enclosed — golf clubs in a bag, a card table in a box — keep them in their original containers, and then put them in a closet, on a shelf, or on the floor as befits their size. Though original boxes are great for storage, keeping empties is a waste of space. Do you need the box for the water glasses in your kitchen cupboard? Nope! The no-empties rule has two exceptions: boxes for electronic equipment (computers, VCRs, CD players, and the like), which you'll need along with the foam packing inside if you ever have to pack or ship your components, and a few empty boxes for shipping gifts. Break down shipping boxes and put them with your gift-wrap center.

* **Containers:** Clear plastic containers in a variety of sizes enable you to group like items and see them clearly. Label each one with its contents for even easier identification. If you have a large family and are storing individual possessions such as clothes or kids' papers, try transparent boxes in different colors. This trick is great for separating boys' and girls' hand-me-down clothes. Mark the sizes on the boxes.

* **Pullout drawers:** From large floor units to minis that sit on a shelf, drawers do the job, too.

☺ ☺ ☹ ☺ ☺ ☹ ☺ ☺ ☹ ☺ ☺ ☹ ☺ ☺ ☹ ☺ ☺ ☺ ☹ ☺

❊ **Coverings:** You can't fit card-table chairs into a pullout drawer but you can store them dust-free by draping them with an old sheet. Even better are the clear plastic drop cloths they sell for covering furniture while painting, which enable you to see what's underneath and look less scary.

After you have everything neatly contained, you'll need a few places for those containers. Because the basement is an area for many diverse activities, you'll want to use wall space to keep stuff off the floor. Keeping the floor clear also lessens the potential for any items to be lost to water damage. For your contained items, sturdy shelves are the next step. Metal shelves like the ones pictured in Figure 12-1 will withstand a flood and hold a lot of weight. Depending upon what you store and the earthquake activity in your area, you may want to secure free-standing shelves to the wall.

Cabinets, by hiding their contents away, make a nice alternative to shelves. Cabinets are suited for smaller items such as office and craft supplies, or chemicals and paints.

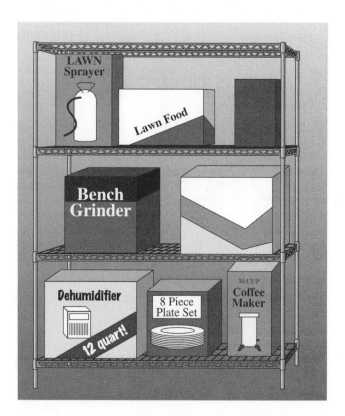

Figure 12-1: Metal shelf units can stand up to plenty of weight and basement weather.

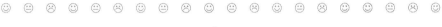
Strategizing your storage solution

You have basement storage principles down; now how can you put them into action? Here are some examples of how you can group items by category, contain them well, and position them for appropriate access in your basement storage area.

- ❋ **Luggage:** Keep only the pieces you use, with larger ones in back and smaller ones in front (don't nest them; you'll forget all about the inside pieces). Try under the stairs if you have space.

- ❋ **Home office:** Store extra inventory and office supplies on shelves and/or in clear containers.

- ❋ **Paperwork and memorabilia:** Keep tax records for the past seven years, real estate papers, wills, warranties, kids' memento boxes (see Chapter 10 on the workspace). Store them on a high shelf to protect them from floods; move indispensable items to a safe-deposit box.

- ❋ **Hobby and craft supplies:** Store extra inventory in clear containers.

- ❋ **Picnic supplies:** Store your cooler, basket, portable dishes and utensils, grill, charcoal, blankets.

- ❋ **Holiday and party supplies:** Stow away decorations, dishes, silverware, a large coffeemaker, a punch bowl, cups, card table, and chairs.

- ❋ **Bulk food and paper supplies:** Store canned goods, drinks, and other nonperishable foods, bath tissue, napkins, and paper towels. Buy in bulk on sale or at warehouse stores, and shelve according to the pantry principles in Chapter 3.

- ❋ **Extra refrigerator and/or freezer:** Store drinks, ice, party overflow, and big-batch recipes on a platform to protect them from fridge floods.

Items you're saving to donate can be collected in boxes or bags until it's time for a pickup or a run to your local charity. See Chapter 2 for more on donating as a great clutter-busting technique.

Basement Activity Centers

Use the center concept to organize basement work and play by activity. Whether you have separate rooms or simply dedicated areas, sectioning off each center and stocking the space with the equipment and supplies you need gives you fingertip management of the task. You can find entire chapters in this book on the family room, playroom, and laundry room, so if any of these are in your basement, browse Chapters 4, 5, or 9,

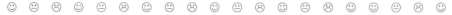
respectively, for how to set them up. Following is the lowdown on creating basement centers for the workshop, crafts and hobbies, exercise, and gift wrapping centers.

The workshop

Happiness central for home improvement nuts but often a source of distress for those who don't know a wrench from a rivet (and would rather not), the workshop can become more useful to every household member with some simple organizational techniques.

Workshop floors often seem unfriendly, with cold, hard cement the default mode and messy activities such as sawing and painting removing the motivation to improve. But take note: Tiling the workshop floor can warm up the room without making it any less washable. Another step up the comfort scale is indoor/outdoor carpet, which cleans up, lasts long, and doesn't mind getting wet.

 Change your life: Get a wet-dry vacuum. Designed to suck up anything from wood shavings to spilled milk, this all-purpose appliance will serve you well in the workshop, kitchen, and car.

Tools

Do you use tools only when you can't get the maintenance man on the phone and there's no handy friend at hand? Then a single toolbox stocked with the basics will do. Here are the basics that everyone should own:

- ❁ Hammer
- ❁ Wrench
- ❁ Four screwdrivers (a big and small each of regular and Phillips)
- ❁ Two pliers (needle-nosed and regular)
- ❁ Nails (all types)
- ❁ Screws (all types)
- ❁ Picture hangers (large and medium — skip the small)
- ❁ Tape measure

 Power tools aren't just for experts and geeks. You can now get cordless, rechargeable, power-driven versions of everything from screwdrivers to drills that make short work of tasks that need tools.

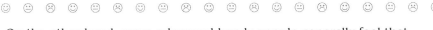

On the other hand, more advanced handy people generally feel that accomplishing all jobs takes various sizes of tools, so the best way to organize the resulting proliferation is to hang them by similar type on a pegboard. From needle-nosed to supersized, put all the pliers together. Screwdrivers are a group, subdivided into regular and Phillips format and arranged by size.

Parts and other small stuff

Swamped with screws, nails, nuts and bolts, and mollies? Get as many sets of clear mini-drawers as you need to give each part its place. Label the drawers to give the visual image written reinforcement.

You may be surprised to hear me say it, but never throw out an unidentified part. If a screw falls from somewhere and you can't find its source, hold onto it and you may locate the empty hole soon enough. Label one drawer "Lost Parts," put the current mystery pieces there, and purge them as they become old-timers.

Supplies: Glues, tape, paint, and light bulbs

There are as many sticky substances as there are things that need sticking together, running the gamut from airplane glue to glue guns. Do you really need them all? Probably not. You can fix most things with an adhesive trio: plastic glue, super glue, and cement glue. Go through your collection and toss anything else you haven't used in a year or that's clogged or dried out.

You also need masking tape, duct tape, and sealing tape for other sorts of sticking; paints and varnishes for surface improvements; and extra light bulbs to replace burnouts throughout the house. Store all these supplies in a cabinet, if you have one; otherwise, use a few containers on a shelf. Old shoeboxes are a low-cost alternative for containing tapes or glues; just be sure to label the outside with the contents so you know where to look. And don't forget to mark the paint cans to indicate which room and wall or ceiling they go with.

The hobby and craft center

Having a hobby is all about fun, so set up a shipshape center that makes every session a pleasure. If the hobby area shares a room with other activities, delineate a center that accommodates equipment, supplies, and work. Do you need wide open space far away from a window to practice your golf swing, or a darkroom to develop photographs? A table to spread out your sewing, or a big piece of floor for a train track? Take space, lighting, and the comfort of your surroundings into account when designing your hobby center.

Next, designate space to store equipment and supplies. Closets, cabinets, or shelves can contain big stuff, such as a painting easel or sewing machine, while free-standing or shelf-top drawers are good for smaller supplies. Storage containers can get quite specialized, so check associations, Web sites, catalogs, and stores dedicated to your hobby for systems targeted to your particular supplies.

There's a cardinal rule for keeping crafts and hobbies organized, one that adults often have an easier time teaching to their children than following themselves: Always, always clean up and put things away at the end of every session. Not only does this prolong the life of your paintbrushes and prevent a passing child or dog from taking a lick, but tidying up also makes coming back the next day a lot more fun.

Exercise center

The sheer weight of exercise equipment and bouncing bodies begs you to locate your workout center in the basement, close to the ground and far away from parts of the house that won't be enhanced by the scent of sweat. But make it nice. The model exercise area is a rejuvenating getaway, a place to leave your workaday worries behind and focus on the pleasures of feeling fit.

Not up for sit-ups on the cement floor? Carpeting can ease your crunches, as well as absorb the shock to your knees if you engage in high-impact activities. Carpet-store remnants can be a cost-effective route to an exercise-friendly floor.

Arrange big equipment to account for the clearance you and any workout partners need for each activity. Folding equipment can create additional space for floor work when not in use. Store smaller equipment such as hand and leg weights, jump ropes, and resistance bands in a box or container sized to the job.

Finish off your exercise center with some entertainment. A mini media center with a portable stereo and/or television can motivate and prolong your workouts, whether you cue up an exercise program, the news, your favorite tunes, or a book on tape.

Keep exercise equipment that you only use outdoors, such as wrist weights for walking, in the closet closest to your exit door.

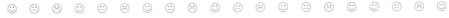

Gift-wrap center

If wrapping a simple gift requires a trip to the attic for paper, a desk drawer for scissors, and the kitchen for tape, you can get back the joy of giving with a gift-wrap center. A single location speeds up the job and also helps you keep inventory and restock supplies, so you're not running late for Sally's birthday party only to discover that you don't have a single sheet of wrapping paper in the house.

You can purchase specially designed plastic containers to hold flat and roll wrap, ribbon, bows, scissors, tape, gift cards, and pens as shown in Figure 12-2. A box about the size of a paper shopping bag is another option for standing rolls on end; put the remaining supplies on shelves or in drawers.

Stock your wrapping center with both birthday and all-occasion paper and trimmings. Holiday wraps can be stored with holiday supplies until the season draws near.

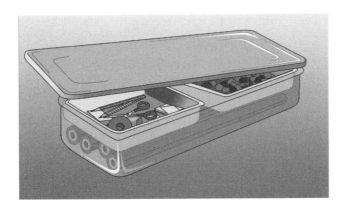

Figure 12-2: Wrapping containers make gift-giving easy.

The Attic

The word alone can conjure up images of cobwebs and junk. Although a cluttered place crawling with spiders can quickly become household Siberia, a well-administered attic can serve as a powerful primary or adjunct storage area — so break out a broom and the five W-A-S-T-E questions and go clean it out.

Attic storage principles are essentially the same as in the basement, except that the place is likely to be hotter in the summer and colder in the winter, which makes the attic a bad choice for photos, tapes, books, and papers that could be ruined by extreme temperatures. Food doesn't fare well here either. However, clothes, toys, decorations, luggage, off-season sports equipment, memorabilia, and many other items do fine in the attic. Refer back to the section on storage earlier in this chapter and make full use of the space under the rafters.

These items work well in the attic:

❀ **Clothes:** Off-season clothes, off-season coats, costumes, and hand-me-downs in waiting, sorted by category as described in Chapter 11.

❀ **Sports equipment:** Off-season or rarely used skis, golf clubs, bikes, racquets and balls, bowling balls, volleyball net, sports shoes, and so on.

❀ **Toys:** To save for younger children or rotate back into active stock (see Chapter 5).

❀ **Baby (when you're not expecting another right away):** Clothes, accessories, blankets, equipment (crib, playpen, carrier, swing), toys, books, CDs, and tapes.

Chapter 13

Out of Sight but Not Out of Mind: The Garage, Patio, and Shed

When you clean up your outdoor spaces, you can get outside with everything you need to have a great time. Spruce up the grass. Throw dinner on the grill. P-L-A-C-E summarizes a plan to patrol your borderlands, putting everything in its place so that you can enter and exit the house with grace.

❀ **Purge:** Toss unused, outgrown, or broken sports equipment and toys, old supplies, and things too dirty or dusty to use.

❀ **Like with like:** Organize items into centers by like type: car accessories and supplies; tools; lawn, garden, and snow equipment and supplies; sports equipment and toys; pool supplies; patio furniture; and grill equipment.

❀ **Access:** Move inside toys back into the house. Keep car supplies on a high shelf out of the reach of children or enclose them in a cabinet. Put off-season sports equipment into indoor storage or the shed. Keep patio furniture and/or lawn and snow equipment in a shed. Put recycling bins near the garage door leading to the house.

❀ **Contain:** Use a cabinet or shelving in the garage for car supplies and a pegboard for tools. Hanging hooks can hold bicycles, lawn chairs, and ladders. Place sports gear into racks and balls and toys into baskets.

❀ **Evaluate:** Can you drive in and out of the garage and park with ease? Is everything you need for outdoor activities here and nothing else? Do the patio furniture and grill set have off-season homes? Does your property appear neat and tidy all the way from the outside in?

Getting a Ground Plan: The Garage

The ground rule for what goes in the garage is that you currently use it there or outside. General storage and off-season equipment can be relocated into the house or storage shed, if you have one. Use W-A-S-T-E (see Chapter 2) to decide what's worth keeping and what's a waste of space.

Before you do anything, move the cars out of the garage, clear everything off the floor, and hose it down, starting at the back and working your way out the door. Sweeping does little more than rearrange dust in the garage. A hose with a good strong stream, on the other hand, can get dirt off the floor and down the driveway. The wet-cleaning method may also provide the motivation you need to keep the garage floor clear.

Next, park your cars in the garage, take a piece of chalk, and mark their width and length on the floor and their height on the wall. Open the doors and mark off their clearance curve. This is the space you need to keep clear as you consider where everything else goes.

Finish off your garage ground plan by figuring out what goes where. Move out the cars, survey the space, and see where you can install each of three options:

- **Hanging hooks:** You can get bikes, big tools, sports equipment, lawn chairs, and ladders off the floor by hanging them on heavy-duty wall- or ceiling-mounted hooks. Put all items in easy reach and reserve the lowest altitudes for the heaviest items.

- **Open shelving:** Whether mounted on the wall high enough to clear the cars or free-standing on the floor, shelves can hold and organize smaller items and supplies like car supplies.

- **Closed cabinets:** They may cost more than open shelves, but cabinets can save time and work by keeping their contents clean.

Think vertical in the garage. There's lots of wall space above automobile level just waiting to get used.

Dealing with Your Wheels: The Car Center

In today's mobile society, few investments yield such tangible benefits as a car. Often serving almost as second homes, cars take people to work and school, carry home the groceries, provide party transport, expedite

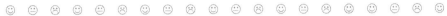
errands, and enable trips near and far. With all these roles to play, cars can fall victim to wear and tear if not cared for and maintained. Protect your investment with organizational tactics that keep your vehicles in drive.

Parking without wrecking

How often do you hit a garbage can or level a bike when pulling into or out of the garage? Ease the parking process by purchasing a plastic parking guide that tells your tires just where to stop. If you're the more playful type, you may prefer to hang a tennis ball from the ceiling that taps your windshield to tell you that you went far enough. Trick number three is a chalk or pencil mark on the wall. When your shoulder is even with the line, shift into park and power down.

 Try backing into your spot. Not only can this position the trunk closer to the door to the house for loading and unloading, but when you leave again you can exit the garage with a clear view of kids playing and cars driving by.

Supplies for a smooth ride

Unless you're a car-wash junkie and mechanic's addict, you probably want some supplies on hand to keep your ride running and looking smooth. The list for the average motorist includes

- Antifreeze/coolant
- Windshield wiper fluid
- Motor oil
- Soap
- Bucket, sponges, and old towels
- Upholstery protector
- Fabric cleaner
- Whitewall tile cleaner
- Rubbing compound
- Wax
- Touch-up paint
- Squeegee
- Chamois cloth
- Extra windshield wipers
- Extra air filters (you can easily change them yourself)

129

☺ ☺ ☹ ☺ ☺ ☹ ☺ ☺ ☹ ☺ ☺ ☹ ☺ ☺ ☹ ☺ ☺ ☺ ☹ ☺

Keep all these precious but poisonous supplies on a high shelf out of reach of passing children. If you wash your own car, you may want to contain your drying towels in two small garbage cans — one can for clean towels and one for dirty, until you have enough to wash.

Maintenance is made easy by hanging a bulletin board on a garage wall to post a spreadsheet (like the one in Table 13-1) for each car. One glance can tell you when your car is due for an oil change or tune-up, or whether your mechanic is trying to resell you the same job he did last year. For the full scoop on preventive maintenance tips, check out *Auto Repair For Dummies* (published by Wiley).

> If you like to look under the hood, get a flashlight with a hook designed to hang inside and leave your hands free to work.

Table 13-1 Vehicle Maintenance Checklist

Make: _____ Model: _____ Year: _____

Task	Date Performed	Next Needed
Oil change		
Tire rotation		
Check tire pressure		
Check air filter		
Clean fuel system		
Get tune-up		

Fixing It Neatly: The Tool Center

An avid carpenter or handyperson may prefer a workshop in the garage, where air and sunshine are plentiful and messes aren't a problem, to a basement location. If you're one of these and live in a moderate climate, set up your main workbench here. Part-timers can get by with a pegboard in the garage to hold tools for the cars, bikes, and outdoor equipment, as well as a very long extension cord and an extra flashlight for everything from poking around under the hood to finding your way in a power outage.

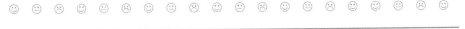

 Stock duplicates of tools you use in the garage and other parts of the house, so you don't have to traverse the property every time you need a screwdriver.

Keep a ladder or two in the garage for high-level jobs. A stepladder can cover most household tasks, while an extension ladder may be required for rooftop adventures. Both can hang on wall-mounted hooks, the stepladder vertically and the tall extension ladder horizontally.

Maintaining the Great Outdoors: Lawn, Garden, and Snow Centers

By organizing the equipment, implements, and supplies you need to keep your lawn neat and green, the garden in bloom, and the winter snow out of the way, you can turn these tasks into stress-busting pastimes.

Start by showcasing this season's equipment. The lawn mower in the summer and the snow blower in the winter get front-and-center placement in the garage, while off-season equipment can be stored out of the way. Begin the season with an annual tune-up of lawn or snow equipment and end it by emptying out the gas. Got multiple gas cans? Label them so you know what fuel is for which machine.

After you have the equipment situation under control, organize your implements well. Group garden tools by like type and hang or contain them so they're easy to take out into the yard. Here are some guidelines:

* Rakes, lawn edgers, shovels, and other large tools can hang from hooks or special holders that grasp the handle with rollers. Put the tool head up rather than down to keep it out of the reach of kids. (This works well for snow shovels, too.)

* Group smaller tools, trowels, spades, hand rakes, and so forth in a bucket that you can use to tote them out to the yard.

* Put planters, starting pots, and bulbs into boxes or plastic dishpans to keep them neat and mobile.

* Keep your garden seeds fresh in the refrigerator until you're ready to plant. A second fridge in the basement is an ideal home for your seed collection.

Bags of dirt, fertilizer, and plant food offer potential snacks to mice, rats, and chipmunks, and flimsy paper containers yield easily to rodents' teeth. Save yourself a mess by storing soil and fertilizer in sealed plastic containers or covered garbage cans.

Spare your back the strain of carrying a big bag of sod or fertilizer by adding a hand truck or wheelbarrow to your lawn and garden routine.

 Keep a bucket of sand on hand to clean off dirty garden implements. Simply dunk the tool, work it up and down a few times, and put the tool away neat and clean. Replace the sand as necessary. If you choose to wash your tools with water instead, dry them well to prevent rust.

Winning Ways to Play: The Sports and Game Center

Whether you live for tennis or you like to go by trike, playing outside is an all-ages pleasure, and the equipment involved can create all-ages clutter. Skis going every which way, balls underfoot, jumbles of toys, and bicycle traffic jams can clog the garage and make play a chore. Tackle your sports and recreational gear with organizing systems that can restore order to all your outdoor fun.

Sports racks are great no matter what your game is. From balls, bats, and rackets to bikes, golf clubs, snowboards, and skis, you can find a rack for every sport. You can be on the greens like greased lightning or head for the courts with a clear mind when you keep your equipment neat in an organizer designed for the job. For larger equipment, overhead hooks can stow your gear up and out of the way. Wall or ceiling hooks can hold bikes, sleds, and a variety of equipment. The trick is that high-hanging hooks are hard to reach, especially if the equipment is heavy, so consider swapping the location of bikes and sleds by the season.

And of course, you want to contain everything. Containers are great for those smaller pieces of equipment. Sort smaller equipment and toys into containers by type. A basket can hold balls and Frisbees, squirt guns could go into a bucket, and jump ropes can hang on a wall hook to keep them tangle-free.

 Buying your first swing set? Select one that can grow with your children, with accessories that can easily be replaced as they move from fire poles to parallel bars.

The Trash and Recycling Center

Trash management begins at the source, so start by compacting garbage as much as you can. Whether you use a mechanical trash compactor, your

132

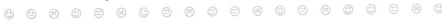

own hand around a soft metal can, or an old-fashioned downward push to wastebasket contents, you can save space and reduce the number of trash-toting trips by maximizing its density.

Keep a recycling container — an official bin or a more attractive trash can — alongside the kitchen wastebasket for all your plastic, glass, and cans. Make sure the recycling bin looks different from the wastebasket so you don't get confused.

Contact your local waste disposal company to find out where and when to dispose of hazardous materials such as used motor oil, old cans of paint, and batteries. Some automotive stores will take your old car batteries for recycling.

 If you live in an apartment, without the luxury of a garage, you can still be eco-friendly. Keep two brown paper bags alongside the kitchen wastebasket to contain paper and other recyclables, respectively. As they fill up, take them down to your building's recycling center or to your car trunk to tote them yourself.

Ideally, garbage cans and recycling bins go right inside the garage, with the newspaper bin in the prime spot for daily pitching. Post a list of recycling rules on the wall to help you meet any sorting requirements.

 If you do yardwork, dedicate a separate can or two to lawn and garden trimmings and keep the garden cans in the yard closest to their use for the sake of convenience. If you have no out-of-the-way spot to place them, install a small decorative fence to block their view.

The Patio or Deck

Move anything you're not using at least weekly to the garage, shed, or basement. Next, group like items together. These may include the following:

* Grill equipment and supplies, outdoor tableware

* Citronella candles, insecticides, insect repellants

* Patio furniture, cushions, and accessories

Finally, contain all the items in a deck storage box. A deck box can keep everything you need — cushions, croquet set, outdoor tablecloth, and so on — in reach yet out of the elements.

Apartment or condominium patios and balconies

In multiresident units, a small patio or balcony is often all the great outdoors you have. If so, the balcony may hold everything from a bicycle and beach chairs to a small potted garden to a barbecue grill and table. If you store things on your balcony, be aware of the view you present to your neighbors. If you wouldn't want to look at your mess, chances are the neighbors would rather not either. Try a deck storage box to keep a few things out of sight.

Lightweight patio furniture that folds is easiest to take outside for a good cleaning under a hose or spigot. If moving furniture for cleaning is too cumbersome, try a spray cleanser and damp cloth. Another option is to use a bucket of soapy water and a second bucket of clean water for rinsing, just like washing your car.

Patio furniture

You want patio furniture to be comfortable, durable enough to weather outdoor living, and easy enough to haul back into the garage or shed when winter approaches. Buy folding versions of chairs, tables, and lounges for easy off-season storage; choose heavy-duty weatherproof models for frequent use. Put the cushions away every night in the garage, storage area, or deck box to keep them clean and dry. To keep the patio area looking nice and free of cobwebs, hose down furniture kept outside once a week. If you have portable chairs for picnics or the beach, store them on hooks in the garage or in the storage shed.

The grill center

Longing to light up the barbie? Organize everything you need to get the fire started. Here are a few hot tips:

* If you have a gas grill and a source of gas in the house, consider installing a direct connection so you don't have to refill the tank.

* Contain charcoal in a covered plastic garbage can next to the grill. Use rubber gloves to handle charcoal without turning your hands black.

* Keep fire-lighting materials on a high shelf in the garage. Starter cubes or electric lighters are more environmentally friendly than lighter fluid.

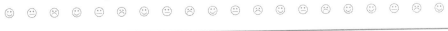

Don't ever light a grill inside the garage or house.

Clean out the grill at the start of the season, checking tubes and vents for cobwebs and debris that could turn into fire hazards. Each time before you light up, give the grill rack a scrub with a grill brush to remove any dirt that's landed there since the previous use. Repeat after you're done cooking and the fire has died down to clean off cooked-on food and grease. If you use charcoal, empty the ash after each cooking session to keep it from blowing all over the yard and to give you a clean start next time. Turn the faux briquettes in gas grills a few times a season to burn off the grease.

The Storage Shed

A storage shed alongside the house is quite handy for keeping outside equipment such as the snow blower or lawn mower, garden tools and supplies, and even bikes if the structure is big enough. If you have a shed full of junk right now, go throw the stuff away and discover your garage annex.

Follow the principles of P-L-A-C-E in the storage shed, maximizing access by placing the most frequently used items in front and enclosing items in containers by like type. Install a shelf or two to contain small items and hooks for rakes and tools. Put all the hooks on one wall, so you aren't watching your head on both sides of the shed.

☺ ☺ ☹ ☺ ☺ ☹ ☺ ☺ ☹ ☺ ☺ ☹ ☺ ☺ ☹ ☺ ☺ ☹ ☺

Part 4

Organizing Your Life: Time-Management Tips

Whoever said that time is money was understating the case in the extreme. Time is a part of life itself, and Part 4 can help you make more of every moment.

No matter how smart or how rich you are, you never get more than 24 hours in a day. However, with the right time-management techniques, you can easily add some extra accomplishments or free time. Trim a week off an unwieldy project. Make a plan for five years out; then make your plan come true. The principles in this part can help you put time on your side — at work and at play — to get the most living out of every day, not to mention arrive at appointments early, pick up your kids on time, and make it to the movies before the previews start.

Chapter **14**

Managing the Household Information Flow

In This Chapter

☺ Organizing your information center

☺ Filing your way to freedom

☺ Managing your mail like a pro

From the daily onslaught from the mailbox, to opening the bundles of friendly reminders, homework assignments, and completed projects from your children's school, you're likely inundated with piles of paper each week. This chapter gives you the tools you need to handle all the information that flows your way each day, file the keepers, and free yourself from yesterday's news. You *can* dig yourself out from under those piles of paper and prevent them from happening again. It's a bold promise, but when you discover how to put information in its place, the flow turns from an organizational foe into a very good friend.

The Household Information Center

Your household information center may be located center stage at a built-in desk in the kitchen, in a room all its own, in a corner of the basement (if it's used daily), or it may share quarters with a home office you use for business.

The desk is the heart of the household information center. If you make do with your old kitchen table, buy some freestanding drawers such as those shown in Figure 6-1 in Chapter 6.

Household filing system

Create your home filing system according to the ABC principles. Active files go in a cabinet in the information center, and inactive files should be boxed up for storage. You should be able to contain home files in about two file drawers (unless you have an extensive financial portfolio) plus a box for warranties.

If mounds and piles are your usual MO, try this simple-but-elegant concept: files. Done right, filing is as easy as ABC: activity level, basic tools, and classification and color. Be a filer, not a piler!

Active versus inactive files

What's the difference between a current project file you pull out five times a day and one containing your tax returns from five years ago? Tons! Fingertip management dictates that only your active files should be taking up valuable space near your valuable self. Totally inactive files, such as old tax returns, belong in shadowy spaces where only auditors would dare to tread.

Basic tools you need

If you're a carpenter, you need a hammer and nails, a stud finder, and a leveler. If you work with papers, your tools are binders, folders, hanging files and frames, labels and tabs, and suitable containers to put it all in. Assemble your tools before you start so you can file as you organize.

- **Binders:** Binders make the best holders for papers you refer to like a book: procedure and training manuals, computer information, logs, and reference material.

- **File containers:** Anything that doesn't get bound in a binder needs to be filed in a folder inside a hanging file. That's right — *a file that hangs from a frame.* Places to hang files include drawers, plastic file boxes or crates, and cardboard storage boxes.

- **Hanging files:** Look for standard hanging files, hanging file pockets for larger groupings of files, and label tabs.

- **File folders:** Get the right folder for the right job. Standard folders work great when all the papers are about the same size, but consider *folder jackets* (manila folders with closed sides) when you're worried about smaller pieces and papers falling out.

Classification and color-coding

When you classify and color-code your files, your fingers don't even have to do the walking — your eyes do the looking to find the file you need fast. There are three steps to classifying your files: Choose the main categories, select a system for classifying the files within each category, and make a file index.

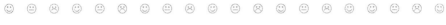

Begin by grouping your files by subject and giving each category a noun for a name. If you have more than ten files in a category, repeat the process to create subcategories. For instance, *Insurance* files could break down into *Disability, Health, Liability,* and *Workers Compensation.*

The most common household filing categories include

- ❋ **Auto:** Keep separate files for each car, including mileage logs, gas receipts (if tax deductible), and maintenance and repair receipts, which can help the resale value.

- ❋ **Career:** Start a résumé file with your first job and keep one copy of each version for reference, with one or two masters showing supervisor names and phone numbers as well as your salary information.

- ❋ **Education:** Save all degrees, continuing education units, certifications, and transcripts. If you have children, keep a file for general information on their schools and year-end (not quarterly) report cards.

- ❋ **Financial:** Keep bank statements in a file. Let the bank store your checks and get a copy if necessary. Retain only the latest utility statements unless you're submitting them for free light bulbs or saving them to create a budget. Keep current tax information in active files. After you finish your annual income tax return, purge anything you aren't required to save and move retained files into inactive storage. The minimum to keep past tax records is seven years, but many experts recommend holding on to returns for life.

- ❋ **Health:** If you currently follow an exercise or diet regime or a course of treatment for a particular condition, keep relevant information in this file. Throw away anything that doesn't pertain to your present condition, because such information changes quickly.

- ❋ **Insurance:** Keep all receipts and insurance-claim paperwork for one year unless the claim is still open.

- ❋ **Legal:** This includes marriage and birth certificates, divorce papers, adoption papers, car titles, passports, real-estate closings, trusts, wills, leases, and so on. Keep copies in your files for reference and store the originals in a safe-deposit box.

- ❋ **Medical:** At the end of the year, transfer medical information to one list per person, including major illnesses and injuries, date, doctor's diagnosis (with name and phone number), and treatment. You can create a computer spreadsheet or word processing table to make tracking medical information easier.

- ❋ **Real estate:** This includes information on your home and improvements. File current home-improvement projects in the active files; put completed home improvements in the inactive files.

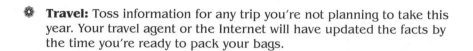
❋ **Travel:** Toss information for any trip you're not planning to take this year. Your travel agent or the Internet will have updated the facts by the time you're ready to pack your bags.

Have you heard about establishing boundaries? Make some in your filing system by keeping all business and personal files separate. Storing personal information at work, where the wrong eyes may run across a private matter, is asking for trouble. If you work at home, a clear distinction between the two types can help you with everything from doing tax returns to pulling the right file when you have a client on the phone.

After you categorize, it's time to classify. You may classify files alphabetically, chronologically, geographically, numerically, or by subject. Choose from these five main classifications according to the contents of the files.

Then, in a database, spreadsheet, or word processing table, make a list of all your files by category, subcategory, file name, and location. Keep your index handy and update it as you add and purge files. Whether you're looking for something or wondering where to put a new piece of paper, you have a one-stop, easy-scan map of your system. Table 14-1 shows how simple your file index can be.

Table 14-1 File Index

Category	Subcategory	File Name	Location

Children's papers and memories

Swamped by small masterpieces of art and literature? Nobody generates more paper than children in school, and viewing each one as a treasure is natural for the creators and their proud parents. The solution? A memory box.

To make a kid's memory box, purchase a file storage box with built-in handles, one for each child. Label it with the child's name. Inside goes one manila folder per year, labeled with the year and containing one drawing, poem, story, book, and writing sample. At the end of the school year, sit down with your child and have him or her pick out the best item in each category to save. There are three simple rules of the game:

☺ ☺ ☹ ☺ ☺ ☹ ☺ ☺ ☹ ☺ ☺ ☹ ☺ ☺ ☹ ☺ ☺ ☺ ☹ ☺

- ✱ You can't keep anything that can crumble or break, which includes artwork with big clumps of paint.

- ✱ Food products such as the ever-favorite macaroni necklace are forbidden. (Not only are they fragile, but food can bring on the bugs.)

- ✱ A child's memento collection cannot outgrow the box. If the box gets full, some old things have to go to make way for the new.

Adding to the memory box makes a nice wrap-up to the school year and teaches the lesson that less is more. Now whisk that box off to a storage area for lesson number two: Living spaces aren't for archives.

Junior-high and high-school papers

Junior-high and high-school kids need a functional filing system to track their schoolwork and papers pertaining to activities. Give teens a head start on high achievement by teaching them to manage information flow from the get-go.

To set up a junior filing system, buy a sturdy container, such as a crate, with a built-in rack for hanging files. Use hanging file folders and tabs to create general categories for academics — math, science, social studies, history, foreign language, arts, and so on. Stick to generic names so you won't have to rename the category each year as the child segues from algebra to geometry. Add activity categories such as sports, clubs and groups, lessons, religion, and so forth, and one more for school information.

Mastering Your Mail

First, understand that mail time is not when the mail comes — mail time is when you choose. The best strategy is to set an off-peak time for opening mail every day and stick to it as much as possible. Whether e-mail or snail mail, remember that the mail doesn't control you; you control the mail.

Smooth mail management calls for quickly sorting and whisking each item to the appropriate file or to the trash, and you can take your first pass without even opening an envelope. R-A-P-I-D is the road to a fast first response to the mail.

First assemble your mail-processing tools: a letter opener (why risk paper cuts?), your calendar/organizer, a highlighter, and date stamp if you use one. Take your stack of unopened envelopes and sort your mail into the following five piles.

☺ ☹ ☹ ☺ ☺ ☹ ☺ ☺ ☹ ☺ ☺ ☹ ☺ ☺ ☹ ☺ ☺ ☺ ☹ ☹ ☺

- ❀ **Read:** Newsletters, catalogs, reports

- ❀ **Attend:** Notices for meetings, workshops, conferences, perform-ances, events, store sales

- ❀ **Pay:** Bills (window envelopes are a clue)

- ❀ **Important:** Memos, correspondence, and anything you can't iden-tify (presume important until proven otherwise)

- ❀ **Dump:** Junk — ads, solicitations, political flyers, and so on (don't even open these — just toss)

 If one of the pieces of mail is another invitation for a credit card you don't want, rip right through the unopened envelope before throwing it away. This prevents someone else from signing the form, saying you moved, and run-ning up a tab on your dime.

When you complete your initial sort, open one pile at a time, highlighting important information and entering dates in your calendar as you go. Apply the five W-A-S-T-E questions to each piece and toss what doesn't pass the test. Finally, take the survivors and delegate them, place them in your "take action" file, or file them in your permanent system.

Chapter 15

Getting the Right Job Done and When: Goals and Prioritizing

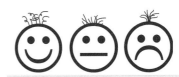

Time isn't money — time is the stuff of life itself. No amount of money in the world can buy a minute or an hour. Don't bother trying to cash in your mutual fund to recover a moment you missed, whether it's a kid's soccer game, a partner's spontaneous kiss, or a meeting that determined the promotions list. Planning means allocating one of life's precious commodities — time — unrecoverable and ever ticking by. Plan today to make tomorrow everything you hope and dream for, or at least to make sure you get the laundry done.

A plan is a road map to get you from here to there — from morning to night, from the beginning to the end of a project, from your first paycheck to a fat investment portfolio. Planning is the same process you go through when you drive to a new destination, though many plans are more important and so promise bigger payoffs than mapping your route across town.

Whether you use time-management techniques to make more of your workplace skills, to free up time for fun, to run your household more smoothly, or simply to maximize the moment, the benefits of planning your day are cumulative, so you want to get started now. Planning may sound like work, but guess what? It's a lot less work than not planning. Furthermore, you can make plotting your course easy with a four-step method to foresee the future. Just follow four steps with the aid of an easy-to-remember acronym — P-L-A-N — which stands for prepare, list, act, and notice.

Preparing for Your Future

Preparation is the part of planning in which you figure out what you're trying to accomplish and why; who will be involved; and where, when, and how you can do it. To help you through the heavy thinking are these high-performance prep questions: the Five Ws plus How. Every time you need a plan, simply ask yourself: Why? What? When? Who? Where? How? The answers can map your path.

Assessing your values

Why? Every plan is driven by values. From deciding on a vacation destination to funding a capital renovation, from buying a home to building a skyscraper, knowing your purpose is the first step to preparing your plan.

Purpose is derived from values, whether held by an individual or an organization — so start your preparation by assessing your values or those of your family. Your answer may be quite different depending on whether you're drawing up a five-year plan or starting a single project or job, whether you're deciding on the kids' activities for the year. You may want to ask yourself some deep personal questions, such as: Is this a time to lead or serve others? Do you want power and the responsibility that comes with it, or would recognition for a job well done please you more? Does financial security take first priority, or is it time to take some creative risks? Take out a piece of paper and write down the top ten values guiding this plan, and then rank them by number. Use Table 15-1 to get started.

When you understand your value structure, write a mission statement to point you to the plan you want to undertake. Mission statements are value-based and answer the question, "Why?" Here are a few examples:

❀ To enjoy some quality time with my mate or significant other.

❀ To have more relaxation time, entertain friends more often, and eat more healthily.

Table 15-1 Assessing Your Values

____ Accomplishment	____ Adventure	____ Caring
____ Comfort	____ Creativity	____ Excellence
____ Family	____ Financial	____ Friendship
____ Fun	____ Happiness	____ Health
____ Home	____ Honesty	____ Humility
____ Independence	____ Knowledge	____ Leadership

☺ ☺ ☹ ☺ ☺ ☺ ☺ ☺ ☹ ☺ ☺ ☹ ☺ ☺ ☹ ☺ ☺ ☺ ☹ ☺

_____ Love	_____ Loyalty	_____ Peace
_____ Power	_____ Recognition	_____ Religion
_____ Security	_____ Serving others	_____ Solitude
_____ Stability	_____ Structure	_____ Trust
_____ Wisdom	_____ Other: _____	_____ Other: _____

Discovering your goals

What? Now that you know why you're making a plan, what are you trying to accomplish? If values are the planning environment, goals are the product — the carrot, the target, the end result or outcome you're aiming for. Are you getting up and going to work every day without a goal? Your lack of direction may cause you to miss out on opportunities for promotion, personal growth, and a comfortable retirement. Trying to improve your tennis game? You may be much more motivated if you set a goal of having a smash serve by August.

Goals can be short or long term, and successful people establish both. Goals can come from you or from a parent, boss, or partner. Effective people balance self-generated with external goals. Setting goals enables actual desires to define the way we spend time — the ultimate empowerment.

Setting goals by the clock

Timing is everything. Start too late on your goals and you won't have time to realize them. Set goals when you're overworked, overwhelmed, tired, or depressed, and chances are they won't represent your truest hopes or best potential. But set your goals when you feel good and can enthusiastically imagine feeling even better, and you're likely to aim high while still being realistic.

Going away to set your goals

Have you ever noticed how going away on a trip can put everything into perspective? How offsite meetings can spark good ideas and build consensus? Getting out of your usual environment can open up your mind to set goals.

Nine types of goals

There are nine main areas to consider when thinking about your goals. If you're doing your annual goal session, you may want to cover them all. Working on a specific plan may keep you within a single category. If it's big goal-setting time, use Table 15-2 to get started.

Table 15-2 Identify Your Goals

Business	Family	Financial	Home	Mental

Personal	Physical	Social	Spiritual	Other

Goal-setting techniques

Now how to decide on your goals? Choose from the following five techniques, or mix and match.

❋ **Six months left to live:** The doctor has just told you that you have six months left to live. What would you do with your remaining days? I know it's morbid, but imagining that your life is almost over is a powerful way to focus on what you want. Try to write down what you'd do in that limited time frame.

❋ **Write your own eulogy:** While you're at it, imagine what you'd like people to say about you after you're gone. Specifically, pick three people — a family member, a friend, and a business or community associate — and write what you'd like to hear, with angel ears, at your own funeral. Compare this with what they may say today. The difference constitutes your goals.

☺ ☺ ☹ ☺ ☺ ☹ ☺ ☺ ☹ ☺ ☺ ☹ ☺ ☺ ☹ ☺ ☺ ☹ ☺

❋ **Likes and strengths, dislikes and weaknesses:** A lighter approach to assessing where you are and what you want in life or a specific situation is to divide a piece of paper into four quadrants and answer the following questions: What do I like/want to do? What do I dislike/not want to do? What are my strengths? What are my weaknesses?

Things you like to do and strengths are goals or components of goals. Things you don't like to do and weaknesses are goals in a different way: How can you get these out of your life? For instance, if you like details but hate face-to-face meetings with people, you probably don't want to be a recruiter, salesperson, or publicist. Consider accounting, engineering, or research. Weaknesses can also become goals themselves if you feel correcting them could help you get what you want.

❋ **Brainstorming:** To brainstorm your goals, take a piece of paper and write your mission statement on the top. Now, thinking of ideas as raindrops and, letting them fall fast and hard, write down every thought that comes to mind, no matter how ridiculous or trivial it may seem. Let one idea lead to the next or make random leaps. Don't edit or judge. Just write. After your brainstorming session, you may want to leave your list alone overnight to incubate. Come back the next day with a fresh perspective, review your list, and use it to write your goal or goals.

❋ **Mind mapping:** Similar to brainstorming, mind mapping is an exercise in free association, but here the emphasis is visual. To chart the terrain of your brain, take a piece of unruled paper and turn it sideways (landscape). In the center, write a keyword or phrase from your mission statement and draw a horizontal oval around it. As that idea sparks new ones, draw branches that are spokes radiating out from the central oval and write them down at the branches' ends. Continue branching from any thought that sparks a new one, letting your mind wander and your pen or pencil take you wherever the branches want to go, like a river flowing into tributaries and streams. You can add pictures or symbols if you like — whatever it takes to make your thoughts visible.

As with your brainstorming list, you may benefit from taking a night away from your mind map, and then coming back and using the map as a guide to writing down your goals.

Achieving your goals

How? Now that you know what you want and have considered the ways to get it, you're ready for the most challenging aspect of procuring your goals in the material world: The mental discipline. An optimistic outlook, keeping lists, remaining undeterred by setbacks, and aiming high all require perseverance and discipline. The rest of this chapter provides concrete tools for achieving your goals. You can prepare your mind to follow through on your plan with the Three Ps: putting it on paper, picturing the play, and pursuing the peak.

Putting it on paper

Studies have shown that people who write things down accomplish them. To-do lists and daily calendars are living proof of this principle. After completing the goal-setting exercises of your choice, write down the final results to complete your commitment and take a load off your mind.

Where you write your goals is less important than getting the writing done, but do choose a place that works for you. Some people like to use the goals section in their daily planner. Others prefer to devote a small notebook to their goals so they have a record over time. You can also write goals on regular sheets of paper and file them by the nine categories and/or date in a section of your filing system, or do the same thing on the computer. Consider how often you like to consult and add to your goals, and choose a format you can access accordingly.

Picture it

If you ever participated in a sport, you probably heard your coach say "picture the play." If a picture is worth a thousand words, visualizing the winning move can be worth its weight in gold.

 Imagine yourself living your goal — in color. See the clothes you're wearing, the way the light falls, the people around you. If your goal is to ski down a mountain, include every inch of snow-covered slope, from the top over all the moguls to the final snowplow at the base. If visualizing from scratch leaves you staring at a blank screen, try clipping pictures from magazines that relate to your goals. You can paste them into a book or divide them into files by topic. If you visualize yourself as you want to be, you can ultimately stop seeing and start being.

Pursuing the peak

No one runs half a race, climbs half a mountain, or pulls her money out of a CD halfway to maturity, so never make a halfway goal. Aim for the top.

Sure, you may face failures and setbacks, obstacles to conquer, and hurdles to clear as you work for your goal. The trick here is to see them coming. What can you do to get the information or training you need to succeed? Take a class? Read a book? Find a mentor or join a support group?

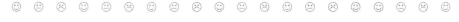

Electricity wasn't discovered in a day and Abraham Lincoln lost eight political races before attaining the nation's highest office. Reach for the top and don't stop until you get there. The pursuit of the peak sets the winners apart from the losers.

You and your plan participants

Who? Every plan involves people. Who are the players in yours?

The first question is what role you play in relation to this plan. Are you acting as a parent, partner, employee, colleague, caretaker, manager, friend? Everyone plays multiple roles. Your mission statement can guide you to yours.

Next consider whose cooperation and support you need to make this plan work. How can you get key players — whether your mother-in-law, your boss, or the best caterer in town — on your side?

The planning time frame

When? Time is of the essence in any plan, and part of your preparation is assigning a deadline. Like the guy who runs the race, look for your finish line. Is the quarterly report due on the first of July? Do you need to book a plane ticket in time to take advantage of 30-day advance rates? Would you like to conquer the beginning ski slopes by January so you can move on to intermediate runs before the snow melts?

Once you set a deadline, another question crops up: What are the steps from here to there? That's the time to break down your goal into smaller pieces. You wouldn't eat a whole pie without slicing it up, so break your goals into achievable steps and then put them in order so you simply move from one small task to the next. (The section on lists later in this chapter will help with this.) Slice your goals into bite-size pieces and succeed.

Finding the right place for your plan

Where? Every plan takes place somewhere. Consider the best setting for yours. If you plan to go back to school, do you want to enroll in the local college so you can continue with your job or family life, or is there a better program somewhere else that offers a more valuable degree? Should your effort to expand your customer base focus on existing or new territories? Can scheduling the kids into summer activities close to home work best, or do you want to try sleepover camp or a visit to faraway relatives?

☺ ☻ ☹ ☺ ☻ ☹ ☺ ☻ ☹ ☺ ☻ ☹ ☺ ☻ ☹ ☺ ☺ ☻ ☹ ☺

Lists You Can Live By

With your preparation in place, turn all those thoughts into lists to guide your actions. Lists are the primary tool for effective time management, and if you haven't discovered their true power, prepare to be pleasantly surprised.

The Master List

Start with your Master List, a comprehensive reference for everything you need to do, present and future, personal and business. You can choose from three main Master List formats:

❀ A 3-x-5-inch spiral notebook

❀ The notes section of your paper organizer

❀ A computer (desktop, laptop, or handheld)

To pick the format that works best for you, consider how you like to arrange and add to your list. The basic concept is that as you think of something new to do, now or later, write it down. This could be a spontaneous thought.

Some people keep their Master List in the order that things spring to mind. Others prefer to organize their list by category or project, starting a new page for each. Some prefer the portability and easy access of paper over the computer, while others like the power to move things around offered by a computer program. For instance, if you decide you want to plant roses but it's the middle of winter, you can easily create a new seasonal section right where you want it. If an upcoming conference starts out as one entry on your Master List but gradually accumulates additional items, you can move them all into one section to find them fast. Still, if your computer isn't on most of the time, are you really going to boot it up to record your midnight inspiration? If not, paper is preferred.

 Whatever form your Master List may take, the important thing is that you write down everything that you need or want to do, in all aspects of your life. It doesn't really have to be organized. That comes next.

The To-Do List

The To-Do List puts your Master List into action on a daily basis. Again, you can keep this on paper or in a computer. Many organizers, both paper and electronic, have a separate spot for your To-Do List. You may like to keep your To-Do List there, or simply use your organizer for appointments and put your To-Do List on a separate piece of paper.

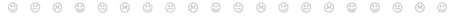

Here are the four steps to creating and maintaining your To-Do List:

1   Create your To-Do List from the Master List.

Today, take about five to ten items from the Master List that you need or want to accomplish tomorrow and write them on your To-Do List. Some of these items may be due tomorrow, while others are intermediary steps or parts of longer-term projects. Don't schedule more than you can handle in a single day after you account for appointments. (There's more on choosing items for your To-Do List coming up.)

2   Rewrite your To-Do List at the end of each day.

The To-Do List, a daily tool, needs to be rewritten every day — not just copied over again. Go back to your Master List and see what's most important for tomorrow. Consider your appointments and errands. Keep your To-Do List fresh and to the point.

3   Set realistic time frames.

Most people tend to overestimate the time required to complete small jobs and underestimate large ones. With this in mind, set realistic time frames for each task on your list. If you did the job before, how long did it take? If it's a new job, jot down how long the task actually takes when you're done so that you know for next time.

4   Allow for interruptions and overflow.

Things happen, so even the most realistic time frames need a cushion to account for interruptions and the unexpected. Double or add a half-hour to each task on your list to account for everything from emergencies to phone calls to cappuccino runs.

Establishing priorities

After you have your rhythms and routines down, prioritize. A priority is a grade of importance plus urgency that determines when you tackle tasks. Here are two ways to assign priorities to your lists:

- ❀ **Numeric rank:** The most thorough prioritizing system is a numeric rank. You hardly want to rank every item on your Master List every night as you prepare tomorrow's To-Do List. But if you already have a rough, priority-based idea of the five to ten items you want to accomplish, simply write them in priority order, ranked from number one to the end.

- ❀ **A-B-C:** If you prefer not to sweat the small distinctions between priorities, try the simpler A-B-C system for ordering tasks: A is for high-priority items, B is for medium priority, and C is for low priority items (but ones that still need doing — otherwise, cross them off the list!) The A-B-C system provides a nice code for your To-Do List, so you can see, at a glance, the grade that you assigned to this task. Is it right for right now?

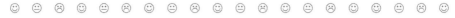

Priorities don't dictate the *order* in which you should tackle tasks, but they do determine *when*. You can probably guess that you don't just go one to ten, or A to C from the beginning to the end of the day. Match the priority to the productivity of the time slot, for example:

- ❀ **Peak time:** A's, possibly some B's, and number one to three priorities
- ❀ **Off-peak time:** B's, C's, and lower priorities such as eight to ten

Calendars

So you prioritized your To-Do List. Now you have to juggle those tasks with commitments from meetings to mom-and-me groups, from doctor's appointments to dinner parties, from baseball games to business lunches. This is where your calendar comes in.

Four types of time

Many people only think to mark specific things they must do or attend in their calendar, but remember, this is a planning tool for your whole life. Use your planner to plot out all your time, not just your appointments, meetings, and parties.

There are four types of time to enter on your calendar. Write the items in order by type as you plan your day, week, or month:

- ❀ Specific appointments, meetings, events, deadlines, trips, visitors, and so on
- ❀ Quiet time
- ❀ Family time
- ❀ Personal time

Schedules change all the time so keep yours looking neat by using a correction pen to white out cancelled or changed entries. It looks much better than scratch marks and frees up the space to write something in its place. I recommend saving your pencil for other purposes, because lead can smudge and become unreadable on the calendar page.

Marking your time in space

Take advantage of your calendar's visual layout to position events in time. If an appointment or meeting falls in the morning, put it toward the top of the day's box. If you plan to go to the gym after work, write it after all of your workday obligations. The idea is to see the flow of your day, week, or month visually.

Depending upon the format of your planner, you may have hours printed on the page. Use these as a guide, even if you approximate (it may not

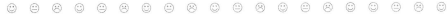
matter exactly what time you get to the gym, unless you're taking a class). Write or circle precise times.

Color-coding your calendar

Color can help you navigate your filing system (see Chapter 14), and make sense of your schedule in a single glance. Choosing a color for each type of event in your calendar can guide your eye to what you're looking for and help you see how well you're balancing the way you choose to spend time. In Table 15-3 is a suggested color scheme.

Table 15-3 A Color Code for Your Calendar

Color Pen	Type of Event	How To/Why
Blue or black	Business (household business if you're a homemaker)	Think B for blue or black and business.
Red	Important events or projects meeting, end of a fundraiser	Neighborhood garage sale, PTA
Pink, green, purple, brown, and so on	Personal	Your favorite color! Match it to your Personal file color. Use a different color for each child.

Using your To-Do List as a planner

If you work primarily on projects, at home or at the office, and you don't need to plan a dozen meetings or appointments, this simple To-Do List may be all you need besides a monthly appointment calendar. Here are the six categories to make up your list:

❀ **To write:** All correspondence, reports, proposals, and so on.

❀ **To call:** All your outgoing calls for the day, including phone numbers, so you can simply dial one after the other.

❀ **To attend:** Meetings, appointments, performances, games, including the time.

❀ **To go:** Errands such as the grocery store or dry cleaner, the library, a sick friend's house, the copy center, and so forth.

❀ **To purchase:** Enter the item and the name of the store so you know just where to go and what to look for when you get there.

❀ **To do:** Everything else that doesn't fall under one of the other five categories.

Keep the categories in this order on a steno pad or something about 6 x 8 inches. As always, rewrite your To-Do List daily, accounting for new priorities and progress down your path.

Chapter 16

Making the Most of Your Personal Time

Progress is a funny thing. With every new invention for doing things faster and better, people just accumulate more obligations and commitments rather than additional free time. You have to keep up to speed on the speediest way to do things just to stay in place. If you actually want to have more time to enjoy your life, you need to be crafty indeed. This is a shortcut chapter jam-packed with ideas for making the most of the time of your life.

Many people have a hard time getting organized because carving out the five minutes here, the hour there, or a weekend afternoon needed to start the systems presented in this book can be tough. The quick and easy tips in this chapter can help you create those windows of time by expediting tasks more efficiently. Line up a few together, and you have an hour to start your filing system.

Getting Out of the House

For most people, mornings aren't peak time for clear thinking, so simply getting out of the house can be one of the day's most daunting jobs. You can take the rigor out of rise and shine by planning your morning just like a project. With a morning plan, everything can go smoothly when you need to coast along the most, enabling you to glide out the door and meet the challenges of your day. Table 16-1 can help.

Table 16-1 Your Morning Timetable

Activity	Time
Be at your destination:	_____
Subtract: travel time	_____
Leave your house at:	_____
Subtract: time to dress, eat, childcare, pet care, read paper	_____
Wake up at:	_____
Subtract: hours of sleep needed	_____
Go to bed at:	_____

Work walking out the door backward, and you end up with a plan for not just getting out of bed, but for getting into bed the night before. One smooth sweep from today to tomorrow ensures you stay caught up on your sleep.

With your morning plan in hand, do some preassembly to get you out and about without even needing to engage your brain. The night before, get ready for the next day by doing the following:

* **Put everything you need — briefcase (including reading material, files, and organizer), laptop, keys, purse/wallet, audiotapes, umbrella, and so on — by the door you exit from in the morning.** (See Chapter 8 for organizing your entryway.)

* **Plan your clothes the night ahead.** (Organizing your closet according to the principles in Chapter 11 can help.) Check the forecast on the late-night news or the Internet. If you live in a volatile climate, you may want to have two outfits in mind and tune in to the early morning weather report. Know the report time of your favorite radio station so you don't miss the weather while you're in the shower.

* **Keep a clock in the bathroom and set it five minutes fast.**

* **Organize your toiletries, makeup, and hair accessories according to the principles of P-L-A-C-E (see Chapter 6).**

* **Make a morning routine that you follow in the same order every day.**

Shopping and Errands

Setting up shopping and errand routines can save time and regularize your schedule. And with home delivery and the Internet, you don't even have to leave the house to accomplish many acquiring missions. Here are some tips to get your shopping done while the clock is ticking:

❀ **Run all your errands at once to save time and gas.** Block the time out in your calendar and go.

❀ **Run errands on the way to somewhere else.** If the dry cleaner is on the way to work, drop your clothes off in the morning and pick them up on the way home. Think like a map.

❀ **Shop the supermarket only once a week, on the same day.** Need fresh fish? Decide whether a specialty store or the grocery store offers the best time/money tradeoff. Run out of milk? Hit the convenience store *once* — then adjust your quantity in the future.

❀ **Order groceries by phone or online and have them delivered.**

❀ **Have prescriptions delivered to your home, ordering by phone to your local pharmacy, by mail, or through one of the many Web sites.**

❀ **Have dry cleaning delivered.**

❀ **Canvass the neighbors for a teenager who can cut your lawn or shovel your snow.**

❀ **Get a babysitter so you can go out.**

❀ **Have music lessons in your home.**

❀ **Order meals out, whether from a take-out place, a specific restaurant, or a restaurant delivery service.**

Cleaning and Chores

Like many people, you're grateful for vacuum cleaners all but you're still waiting for the technological revolution to make keeping the house clean easier. Meanwhile, here are old-fashioned ways to get household work done fast.

Hiring help or delegating

One way to get the job done is to let someone else do it. From hiring out to tapping family members or cohabitants for help, you can turn to other people to ease your burden of chores. Here are some specifics:

❀ **Hire household help.** This time-honored tradition makes even more sense in the age of families with two working parents. Whether you hire out on a regular (weekly or monthly) or special-occasion basis (parties and holidays), consider professional help for everything from cleaning to catering, babysitting, elder care, gardening, pool maintenance, and snow removal.

159

To determine whether hiring out is cost-effective, determine the time *you* would take (not the time the professional would take) to accomplish the job, multiply that number by what your time is worth per hour, and divide the result roughly in half to account for taxes. If the amount is more than the cost of hiring, you're actually paying less by outsourcing — *if* you spend the time saved doing something productive. But then again, sometimes that's not the point.

✿ **Share with a partner.** The days of strict gender lines for household jobs are long gone. Sit down with your mate and work out who's willing to do what, by dividing up tasks and sticking to them or establishing a chore rotation.

✿ **Share with the kids.** Chores are good for kids! Have a family meeting and schedule jobs appropriate to the age level of each child, such as laundry, meal setup, dishes, cooking, garbage patrol, and errands. Young ones can start by discovering how to pick up toys and crafts, make their bed, and choose their clothing at night as their first time-management assignments.

What you can do in the house

When the job of household cleaning falls to you, find the time by setting up routines and planning ahead. Some suggestions include the following:

✿ **Plan the same day each week to clean the house.** Depending upon traffic, you can step up to twice a week for a light once-over on the bathrooms.

✿ **Set aside time *before* holidays to polish the silver and clean the china cabinets, dishes, and crystal glasses you'll need.** Nobody needs this stress in full holiday swing.

✿ **Separate laundry into two different washdays — one for clothes, one for towels and linens — to lighten the load on each day.** Use the same days each week.

✿ **Stash a few extra garbage bags at the bottom of your wastebaskets so when you throw away the current one, a new bag is ready and waiting.**

✿ **Choose at least one day a year to purge your household files if file purging isn't an ongoing process.**

What you can do outside the house

Outside appearances (and functions) do count, so organize your regular outdoor tasks with these tips in mind:

☺ ☺ ☹ ☺ ☺ ☹ ☺ ☺ ☹ ☺ ☺ ☹ ☺ ☺ ☹ ☺ ☺ ☺ ☹ ☺

❋ **Clean the garage floor a couple of times a year.** You may like going there much more.

❋ **Keep the cars in shape by posting repair, tune-up, and tire-rotation schedules on the garage wall.** Have a basic mainte-nance check done before each major trip to head off highway disasters. Wash, wax, and even repaint your baby as often as it takes to stay in love. Maintaining the automobile you have is much cheaper than buying a new car.

❋ **Take the snow blower and lawn mower in for tune-ups before their seasons start.** Add these items to your car maintenance schedule so you don't forget.

❋ **Have blacktop driveways resealed once a year.**

Making Time for Your Family

A few good habits can help unite your household and create more quality time together, as well as ease the logistics of managing and caring for a group. Give these ideas a try to sweeten up your home life.

Savoring together time

With family members coming, going, and lining up for the bathroom, some houses feel more like Grand Central Station than a home. The solution is to schedule routine tasks and fun family time so everyone knows what to expect. These togetherness tactics can help:

❋ Make a schedule for the morning to plan bathroom time and break-fast to get everyone out the door.

❋ Eat dinner together with no television and discuss everyone's day. A shared meal is both emotionally important and an efficient time for communication, so make eating dinner together a priority and schedule it in.

❋ Have a family meeting once a week to set up chores or schedules and provide an open forum for everyone to talk about whatever's on his or her mind. Sunday night is often free of other commitments.

❋ Have a family day once a month with a fun group activity — a picnic, sporting event, amusement park, museum, bowling, skating, minia-ture golf, and so on.

❋ Establish a family reading time, a no-TV night, or a game night.

☺ ☻ ☹ ☺ ☻ ☹ ☺ ☻ ☹ ☺ ☻ ☹ ☺ ☺ ☻ ☹ ☺

❀ Stick little notes in little kids' lunch or school bags every so often with "I love you" or "Have a great day." Keep your college students' mailboxes full. Upon your child's high-school and/or college graduation, write her a letter about growing up and the future.

❀ Make time for relatives. They're more precious than you may realize in the course of busy days.

Finding support systems: Kid care

Kids are bundles of energy, fountains of joy — and in need of constant care. Prevent parental burnout with ways to keep children happy and well cared for while you get some well-deserved grown-up time.

❀ Carpool!

❀ Join a playgroup to meet other parents and share ideas and support while the kids amuse themselves.

❀ Drop a child at a park-district program, preschool, or library program for an hour or two so you can have some free time or run errands.

❀ Shop at stores with play areas to keep little ones occupied while you browse.

❀ Find a gym with child care. No more excuses.

❀ Trade babysitting hours with another parent.

Managing Your Health

It seems everybody is managing her own medical care these days, and the job can get overwhelming. Protect the precious asset of your health with a few proactive habits. Here are some to get you started:

❀ Keep a list of all your doctors in your date book, including name, phone number, and type of practitioner. Add all medicines you regularly take, including how much and what they're for. Throw in your insurance policy number and the number to call to authorize procedures and admissions. This is a quick reference for you — and for someone else in case of an emergency. Also, jot down questions here for your doctor as you think of them, so you can discuss them at your next appointment.

❀ Make annual doctor appointments just before your birthday or at the same time each year. This includes general practitioner, dentist, optometrist, gynecologist, and possibly the dermatologist for a mole check.

❀ Schedule school physicals in July so that you're not caught in the August appointment rush and to be sure your child is covered for the full year for any sports.

☺ ☻ ☹ ☺ ☺ ☻ ☺ ☺ ☹ ☺ ☺ ☻ ☺ ☺ ☻ ☺ ☺ ☺ ☺ ☻ ☺

❀ Keep all open insurance claims in a dedicated file so you know to follow up and can pull papers quickly.

❀ Create a medical history for each family member by keeping a running list of major injuries or illnesses such as chicken pox, broken bones, surgeries, and so forth. Pitch the rest of the documentation; no doctor needs to know that you took penicillin for strep throat in 1983.

❀ If you take more than two pills on a daily basis, including supplements and vitamins, get a weekly pillbox. Fill each compartment on Saturday so you can cruise through the week without thinking. Call the pharmacy for a refill when the last week's worth is sorted. Use the drive-up windows at some pharmacies for quick service or have medicines delivered.

❀ Take vitamins and medications at the same time each day. Write it in your planner if you're trying to get in the habit of something new.

Scheduling Physical Fitness

It's never too late to start on fitness and enjoy daily and long-term rewards. There's just no way out — and this is where a well-organized approach to fitness comes into play:

❀ Find a workout buddy to walk, jog, swim, or play tennis with, or make a standing date to meet at the gym.

❀ Do you love watching basketball, baseball, or hockey? Get off the bench and play.

❀ Bike to work to take care of your commute and your workout at the same time. An easy-to-install rack over your rear wheel can hold your briefcase and laptop.

❀ Work out over your lunch hour. You won't have to worry about getting childcare or cutting into your evening, and you'll return to work reenergized and sharp.

❀ Mix up your exercise from one session to the next — running, doing yoga, lifting weights, swimming, kickboxing, biking — for cross-training and to keep from getting bored.

Entertainment and Recreation

In our hyperachieving society, you can easily forget about fun or get stuck in an entertainment rut, so make and keep a list in two categories: things that you know give you pleasure, and new things you want to try (see Table 16-2). Schedule at least one of each into each month. Here are some ideas to get you started:

☺ ☺ ☹ ☺ ☺ ☹ ☺ ☺ ☹ ☺ ☺ ☹ ☺ ☺ ☹ ☺ ☺ ☹ ☺

❀ Make a lunch date with a non-work friend. Invite a small group to gather for dinner at a restaurant. Stage a dinner party with your dream menu, but don't do all the cooking yourself — assign each guest a dish and send the recipe with the invite.

❀ Take up a musical instrument. Sign up for lessons or join a group.

❀ Join a club or take a class to share your existing or potential passion — bowling, golf, bridge, painting, writing, reading, collecting coins, computer gaming, and so forth.

❀ Go to museums or art institutes. Traveling art exhibits are turning out to be the place to see and be seen, while science museums have become highly entertaining, interactive playgrounds.

❀ Go inline skating, ice-skating, horseback riding, sledding, or skiing on snow or water.

❀ Get into the swing of things and go dancing. Salsa, swing, country-line, techno-rave — they all burn calories and boost your mood!

❀ Use your favorite form of entertainment as a reward for a goal achieved.

Table 16-2 Entertainment Ideas

I love to:	I really want to try:

Making Time for Love

You need a To-Do List to expedite your projects, your tasks, and your love life. If love always comes last in your busy life, perhaps you schedule everything but the very thing you live for. Make prioritizing your paramour easy

☺ ☻ ☹ ☺ ☺ ☹ ☺ ☻ ☹ ☺ ☺ ☹ ☺ ☻ ☹ ☺ ☺ ☻ ☹ ☺

by writing up a Love List of all the special things, big and small, that you can do to make the most of your time together. Keep your list on hand for easy reference both for spontaneous moments and for when you're sitting down to plan your week or month. Make time for love, and all the time of your life will be nicer.

❀ **Schedule a date night, especially if you're married or have been together so long that your idea of a night out is in with the VCR.** Follow all the proper steps: Call your partner on the phone and ask him or her out. Make a reservation for dinner. Plan a movie. Get dressed up.

❀ **Send flowers.** This works for both sexes.

❀ **Send a card — cute, funny, flowery, an inspirational poem — for no reason at all.**

❀ **Tuck a love note in your partner's purse or briefcase, or mail the note to your partner's place of work.**

❀ **Have a scavenger hunt to find a rose or a poem.**

❀ **Make a book of gift certificates for items from a hug to a hand-delivered massage to a romantic getaway weekend.** Give it for Valentine's Day or the anniversary of the day you met.

❀ **Put on some sultry music and have a romantic dinner by candlelight at home.**

❀ **Go out dancing, whatever style you like.**

❀ **Rent a romantic video and cozy up on the couch or carpet with a bottle of wine.**

❀ **Go on a picnic and lie around in the grass looking at the sky.**

❀ **Trade off fantasy nights — yours one time, your partner's the next.**

❀ **Share a candlelit bubble bath.**

❀ **Circle the full moon on your calendar and take advantage of the evening to sneak away and sit in a convertible or on a blanket on the grass.** Stare at the stars, bask in the moonbeams, and talk all night!

Ten Storage Tips for Small Spaces

✤ **Review the P-L-A-C-E section for each room in your home as described in Chapters 2 through 13 and purge like crazy.**
Ask the five W-A-S-T-E questions (outlined in Chapter 2) of every item that crosses your threshold.

✤ **Stack and tier — think vertical.**
Most people naturally perceive on a horizontal plane, but that could represent half or less of your available space. Check out Chapters 3 and 7 for details.

✤ **Add shelves on walls and in cabinets and closets.**
Use wooden shelves instead of coated wire racks to aid balance for small items. Even short shelves can help expand floor space.

✤ **Use space beneath the bed.**
A number of containers, both cardboard and plastic, are designed for storing things under the bed. This is the place for off-season clothes and other infrequently accessed storage items.

✤ **Use countertops.**
Only leave things out on the counter if you're truly space-impaired, however.

✤ **Contain with cabinets.**
Install one above your desk for all your office supplies. Add a free-standing unit to the living room to hide your CDs and videos.

✤ **Hang with hooks.**
Install hooks in your closets to hold purses, hats, recycled plastic grocery bags. Put a big one on a patio or balcony wall to hang a bicycle. Whatever your need, consider hooks as a solution.

✤ **Use the backs of doors.**
A number of coated wire racks are designed to hang on the back of doors and double up their function as storage space, including shoe storage, food storage, or hooks for towels in the bathroom.

✤ **Use rolling carts and drawers.**
Every apartment resident should know the art of carting — containing things in a mobile unit that rolls with the punches. Try a microwave cart in the kitchen, a filing cart in the office, or a set of rolling drawers in the bathroom.

✤ **Buy double-duty furniture.**
Who can afford single-use furniture when space is at a premium? Look for drawers, doors, and shelves in every piece you buy so it has a second use as storage.

Ten Tips for Great Garage Sales

❋ **Schedule your sale.**
May through early September is prime garage-sale season all across the country. Consider getting in on the action.

❋ **Consider placing an ad in the local newspaper to bring in eager buyers.**
If you don't want to pay for an ad, just be sure to post signs on major cross streets and all the way to the site of your sale.

❋ **Team up with neighbors to add impact to your garage sale.**
You can advertise on signs and in ads "three homes . . ." or "the block of . . ." and put out plenty of stuff to entice passers-by to stop.

❋ **Start collecting paper and plastic grocery bags as soon as you decide to have a sale so that your best customers have a way to carry their loot away.**
Also assemble as many boxes as you can to use for display.

❋ **Group like items together and get going on deciding how much you want to sell them for.**
Start with a sheet of paper and a general price list: T-shirts $2, pants $3. When you have your list, mark each item with colored stickers.

❋ **Borrow tables from neighbors — long tables, card tables, anything you can tote — the day before.**
Set up the tables in the garage the night before so you're ready first thing the next morning.

❋ **Go to the bank the day before the sale and buy a roll each of quarters, dimes, and nickels, and at least 20 $1 bills.**
Find a covered box to use for cash. Write down your initial change amount on a slip of paper and store it in the box, subtract it from the total to figure your profit at the end of the day. As soon the box hits $50, start taking additional cash into the house.

❋ **Sell toys.**
If your house is in toy overload, target your sale to children and sell only toys.

❋ **Involve the kids.**
Your garage sale should be a family affair. Have the kids handle the money if they're old enough; it's a great mini-lesson in math. Younger children can have a small lemonade stand for customers.

❋ **If your garage sale is two days long, mark things down the second day by putting up a sign: "25% Off!"**
At noon, change the sign to "50% Off!" or "Best Offer!" *Remember:* You're in the business of selling here.

Index

☺ ☺ ☹ ☺ ☺ ☹ ☺ ☺ ☹ ☺ ☺ ☹ ☺ ☺ ☹ ☺ ☺ ☺ ☹ ☺

Index

☺ ☺ ☹ ☺ ☺ ☹ ☺ ☺ ☹ ☺ ☺ ☹ ☺ ☺ ☹ ☺ ☺ ☺ ☹ ☺

Index

continued

173

☺ ☻ ☹ ☺ ☺ ☻ ☹ ☺ ☻ ☹ ☺ ☻ ☹ ☺ ☻ ☹ ☺ ☺ ☻ ☹ ☺

Index

Index

177